DATE DUE

BIRD FLU: THE NEW EMERGING INFECTIOUS DISEASE

BIRD FLU: THE NEW EMERGING INFECTIOUS DISEASE

VIROJ WIWANITKIT

Nova Science Publishers, Inc.

New York

Library of Congress Cataloging-in-Publication Data

Viroj Wiwanitkit.
 Bird flu : the new emerging infectious disease / Viroj Wiwanitkit (author).
    p. ; cm
 Includes bibliographical references and index.
 ISBN: 978-1-60456-238-5 (hardcover)
 1.   Avian influenza. I. Title.
 [DNLM: 1. Influenza in Birds. 2. Influenza, Human.   3. Communicable Disease Control.   4. Disease Outbreaks—prevention & control. 5. Disease Transmission—prevention & control. 6. Tropical Medicine—methods. WC 515 V819b 2008]
 RA644.I6V57 2008
 636.5'0896203—dc22   2007050812

Published by Nova Science Publishers, Inc. ✦ New York

Contents

Basic Information on Bird Flu

Virology of Influenza

The bird flu of avian influenza is a type of influenza. The bird flu virus can cause a respiratory tract infection similar to general influenza. Generally, the influenza virus can be classified into 3 groups: A, B, and C. The classification is mainly based on the difference between nucleoprotein and matrix antigens [1 – 2]. In addition, influenza can also be classified into subtypes depending on hosts (Table 1). Influenza viruses have a spherical shape with an average size of about 1000 A in diameter and consist of an as yet undefined central structure containing the eight negative-sense RNA molecules of the genome in association with the transcriptase required for mRNA synthesis, an abundant nucleoprotein, and an equally abundant matrix protein [3]. This core is surrounded by a membrane derived from the cell surface in a budding process by which newly-formed viruses are released from the infected cell [3]. During infection, cell membranes are modified by the incorporation of newly-synthesized virus membrane proteins [3]. As a result, the released viruses contain exclusively two different types of virus-specified glycoprotein, hemagglutinin and neuraminidase, and a proton channel protein, M2 [3]. As previously said, the influenza viruses possess segmented, negative stranded RNA genomes (vRNA) and are enveloped [4]. The viruses bud from the plasma membrane of many cells, especially the apical plasma membrane of polarized epithelial cells [4]. Complete virus particles are not found inside infected cells [4]. Virus particles consist of three major subviral components, namely the viral envelope, matrix protein (M1), and core (viral ribonucleocapsid [vRNP]) [4]. Various interactions that contribute to virus assembly are described, including interactions between matrix proteins and membranes, interactions between matrix proteins and glycoproteins, interactions between matrix proteins and nucleocapsids, and interactions that lead to matrix protein self-assembly [5]. For viral morphogenesis to occur, all three viral components, namely the viral envelope, M1, and the vRNP must be brought to the assembly site at previously mentioned cells [4]. Finally, buds must be formed at the assembly site and virus particles released with the closure of buds [4].

Table 1. Hosts for each group of influenza virus

Group	Hosts
Group A	Humans, pig, bird, horse
Group B	Humans
Group C	Humans, bird

Influenza group A is widely mentioned in medicine. A subtype classification of influenza group A virus can be performed based on the difference between two main surface antigens, hemagglutinin (H) and neuraminidase (N). There are 16 H and 9 N forms. In humans, the common forms of H are H1, H2 and H3, and the common forms of N are N1 and N2. In a pig, the common forms of H are H1 and H3. In a horse, the common forms of H are H3 and H7. Of interest, all forms of H and N can be seen in birds. Since there are several combinations of different H and N forms, the nomination of influenza virus is revised by the World Health Organization (WHO) [6 – 8]. The present nomination system is set as the following: "group of influenza virus (A, B or C/ city of first isolation / Strain number / year of isolation." In the case that the virus is firstly isolated in an animal, the nomination system will be "group of influenza virus (A, B or C) / animal / city of first isolation /Strain number / year of isolation."

Influenza A and B viruses contain eight negative-strand RNA segments, while influenza C virus contains seven, each of which encodes 1 or 2 proteins [9]. The RNA segments possess untranslated regions (UTRs) at 3' and 5' ends. The UTRs are composed of highly-conserved terminal nucleotides and segment-specific nonconserved nucleotides located adjacent to the open reading frame of the viral RNAs [9]. They are responsible for transcription, translation, and replication of viral RNA [9].

Table 2. Main 8 segmented RNA genome influenza A virus

Segments	Protein products		
	Name	Number of amino acid	Function
1	PB2	759	cap binding, endonuclease
2	PB1	757	RNA polymerase
3	Pa	716	RNA polymerase subunit, proteolysis
4	Hemagglutinin	560	Receptors binding, membranes fusion
Segments	Protein products		
5	NP	498	a part of RNP
6	Neuraminidase	450	Sialidase activity
7	M1, M2	256, 96	Structures of ion channels
8	NS1, NS2	-	Nuclear export factor, interferon antagonist

As previously mentioned, influenza A virus is an RNA virus. Natural sporadic mutation can be detected. The RNA of influenza consists of 8 segmented RNA genomes [10]. The gene assignment for influenza A virus is as follows: RNA segment 1 codes for PB2, 2 for PB1, 3 for PA, 4 for HA, 5 for NP, 6 for NA, 7 for M1 and M2, and 8 for NS1 and NS2 [11]. M and NS genes of influenza A virus, NA, M, and NS genes of influenza B virus, and M and NS genes of influenza C virus encode two proteins [11]. The two main protein products of RNA are H and N surface antigens as previously mentioned. These two surface antigens are the main targets of host immunity.

Molecular Evolution of Influenza Virus

There are two different mechanisms by which influenza viruses might evolve: (a) because the RNA genome of influenza viruses is segmented, new strains can suddenly be produced by reassortment as happens, for example, during antigenic shift, creating new pandemic strains and (b) new viruses evolve relatively slowly by stepwise mutation and selection, for example, during antigenic or genetic drift [12 - 16]. Scholtissek said that influenza A viruses were found in various vertebrate species, where they form reservoirs that do not easily mix [12]. Ina and Gojobori performed a study to examine whether positive selection operates on the hemagglutinin 1 (HA1) gene of human influenza A viruses (H1 subtype) by statistical method [17]. According to this research, for nonantigenic sites, the nucleotide diversities were larger at synonymous sites than at nonsynonymous sites and for antigenic sites, the nucleotide diversities at nonsynonymous sites were larger than those at synonymous sites [17]. Ina and Gojobori suggested that positive selection operates on antigenic sites of the HA1 gene of human influenza A viruses (H1 subtype) [17]. Sugita et al. studied the molecular evolution of hemagglutinin genes of H1N1 swine and human influenza A viruses [18]. According to this work, for both viruses, the rate of synonymous substitution was much higher than that of nonsynonymous (amino acid altering) substitution; however, the rate of nonsynonymous substitution for human influenza viruses was three times the rate for swine influenza viruses [18]. Sugita et al. concluded that the difference in the rate of nonsynonymous substitution between swine and human influenza viruses could be explained by the different degrees of functional constraint operating on the amino acid sequence of the hemagglutinin in both hosts [18]. According to the study of Kanegae et al., the nucleotide sequences of the HA1 domain of the H1 hemagglutinin genes of A/duck/Hong Kong/36/76, A/duck/Hong Kong/196/77, A/sw/North Ireland/38, A/sw/Cambridge/39 and A/Yamagata/120/86 viruses were determined, and their evolutionary relationships were compared with those of previously sequenced hemagglutinin (H1) genes from avian, swine and human influenza viruses [19]. According to this work, the swine strains sw/North Ireland/38 and sw/Cambridge/39, are clearly on the human lineage, suggesting that they originate from a human A/WSN/33-like variant [19]. However, the classic swine strain, sw/Iowa/15/30, and the contemporary human viruses, are not direct descendants of the 1918 human pandemic strain, but did diverge from a common ancestral virus around 1905 [19]. According to the study of Nerome et al., the complete nucleotide sequences of the neuraminidase (NA) genes of two reassortant (H1N2) and two H3N2 influenza A viruses isolated from pigs were determined, and phylogenetic relationships between these and previously reported N2 NA genes were investigated [20]. According to this study, although the rates of synonymous silent substitutions for the swine and human viruses were nearly identical, the rate of non-synonymous amino acid changing substitutions for swine virus NA genes was about 60% of that for the human virus [20].

Endo et al. studied evolutionary pattern of the H 3 hemagglutinin of equine influenza viruses [21]. The study was the first demonstration that multiple evolutionary lineages of equine H3N8 influenza virus circulated since 1963 [21]. Daly et al. studied antigenic and genetic evolution of equine H3N8 influenza A viruses [20]. Daly et al. said that some mixing was believed to occur as American-like viruses had been isolated during outbreaks of equine influenza in the UK [22]. Daly et al. proposed that the cocirculation of two antigenically and genetically distinct lineages of equine influenza H3N8 viruses had serious implications for vaccine strain selection [22]. Lai et al. said that phylogenetic analysis, using the HA1 gene of more recent American isolates, indicated a further divergence of these viruses into three evolution lineages: A South American lineage, a Kentucky lineage, and a Florida lineage [23]. In contrast to human H3N2 viruses, Lai et al. suggested that the evolution of equine-2 influenza virus resembled the multiple evolution pathways of influenza B virus [23]. Maugueera et al. studied the amino acid sequences of the HA1 portion of the haemagglutinin of two equine A(H3N8) influenza viruses isolated in France in 1993 and 1998 to determine their evolutionary relationship with 51 other HA(1) amino acid sequences available in databanks [24]. Manugueerra et al. suggest that equine-2 strains antigenically related to old prototype viruses might cocirculate with the more recent Eurasian and American lineages [24]. In conclusion, Manugueera et al. proposed that it might be necessary to include both strains representative of recent equine influenza variants and an older prototype strain in the current equine influenza vaccines [24].

For avian influenza, although influenza viruses can infect a wide variety of birds and mammals, the natural hosts of the virus are wild waterfowl, shorebirds, and gulls [25]. When other species of animals, including chickens, turkeys, swine, horses, and humans, are infected with influenza viruses, they are considered abnormal hosts [23]. Saurez said that the distinction between the normal and aberrant host is important when describing virus evolution in the different host groups [25]. Kawoka and Webster reported that the evolutionary changes in the HA of H5N2 viruses that occurred during the epidemic implied that a virus (A/Chick/Washington/84) that was isolated 8 months after the last H5N2 virus had been isolated from poultry in Pennsylvania belonged to the family of potentially dangerous H5N2 viruses and was a direct descendent of the virus that spread to Maryland and Virginia [26]. Kawoka and Webster noted that all of the virulent viruses retained the amino acid changes at residues 13 and 69 in the hemagglutinin [26]. Cauthen et al. described the revelation that at least one of the avian influenza virus genes encoded by the 1997 H5N1 Hong Kong viruses continued to circulate in mainland China and that this gene was important for pathogenesis in chickens [27]. Cauthen et al. noted that there was evidence that H9N2 viruses, which have internal genes in common with the 1997 H5N1 Hong Kong isolates, were still circulating in Hong Kong and China as well, providing a heterogeneous gene pool for viral reassortment, which could be related to the possible future pandemic of avian influenza [27]. Saurez et al. said that the sequence comparison of all eight gene segments showed the

Chilean viruses were also distinct from all other avian influenza viruses and represent a distinct South American clade [28]. Saurez et al. proposed that this might be the underlying reason that the recent epidemic of bird flu did not affect South America [28]. However, Spakman et al. said that the H7N3 avian influenza virus found in a South American wild duck was related to the Chilean 2002 poultry outbreak, contains genes from equine and North American wild bird lineages, and was adapted to domestic turkeys [29].

Bird Flu

There are several types of bird flu, as previously mentioned. The author will hereby present significant details of bird flu which have been reported in the literature.

A. H5N2

The H5N2 virus is an important avian influenza. Outbreaks of this avian influenza have been well documented in USA and Italy. The A/Chick/Penn/83 (H5N2) influenza virus that appeared in chickens in Pennsylvania in April 1983. The highly pathogenic A/Chicken/Penn./1370/83 (H5N2) avian influenza virus, which caused 80% mortality in chickens in Pennsylvania, produced only mild transient illness in experimentally infected pheasants, little or no clinical signs in ring-billed gulls and pigs, and no clinical signs in pekin ducks [30]. Wood et al. suggested that if the first H5N2 virus infecting chickens in Pennsylvania originated from waterbirds, changes in host specificity and pathogenicity for chickens and other gallinaceous birds probably occurred during emergence of the Chicken/Penn./83 virus [30]. Wood et al. noted that it was recommended that attention be given in the future to the isolation of domestic poultry from contact with wild aquatic birds [30]. Kawaoka et al. reported that the amino acid change in the virulent strain at residue 13 was the only mutation that could affect a glycosylation site and this is in the vicinity of the connecting peptide [31]. Kawaoka et al. proposed that the loss of this carbohydrate might permit access of an enzyme that recognizes the basic amino acid sequences and results in cleavage activation of the hemagglutinin in the virulent virus [31]. Nettles et al. conducted a wildlife surveillance for influenza viruses in conjunction with the 1983-84 lethal H5N2 avian influenza epizootic in domestic poultry in Pennsylvania [32]. Nettles et al. found that antibodies against H5 or N2 were found in 33% of the aquatic birds tested [32]. Nettles et al. said that the low prevalence of lethal H5N2 avian influenza virus in wild birds and small rodents strongly indicated that these animals were not responsible for dissemination of the disease among poultry farms during the outbreak [32]. Of interest, Cappucci et al. reported that avian influenza virus could be recovered from the yolk, albumen, and shell surface of eggs obtained from naturally infected chicken flocks in Pennsylvania and Virginia [33]. According to this outbreak, the hemagglutinin concentration of beta-propiolactone-inactivated influenza vaccine containing A/Duck/N.Y./189/82 (H5N2) virus was produced and confirmed for its efficacy [34]. Webster et al. said that simultaneous administration of inactivated H5N2 vaccine and amantadine provided protection; therefore, chemotherapy might be useful in the treatment of a highly pathogenic influenza virus outbreak in humans or other animals when used in combination with vaccine [35].

From October 1997 to January 1998, highly pathogenic H5N2 avian influenza viruses caused eight outbreaks of avian influenza in northern Italy [36 - 38]. The first epidemic was caused by a virus of the H5N2 subtype and was limited to eight premises in backyard and semi-intensive flocks [38]. A nonpathogenic H5N9 influenza virus was also isolated during the outbreaks as a result of virological and epidemiological surveillance to control the spread of avian influenza to neighbouring regions [36]. No virological and serological evidence of bird-to-human transmission of the Italian H5N2 influenza viruses was found [36]. De Marco et al. studied influenza virus circulation in wild aquatic birds in Italy during H5N2 and H7N1 poultry epidemic periods [37]. De Marco et al. reported that only five viruses belonging to H1N1, H11N6, and H2N3 subtypes were isolated from ducks; however, the H5 seroconversion observed in one mallard duck at the beginning of 1998 indicated that H5 virus circulation also occurred in the study area [37].

B. H7N1

H7N1 is another important avian influenza. H7N1 is a cause of many previous avian influenza outbreaks among avian species. The situation in Italy is well known. From the end of March to the beginning of December 1999, an epidemic of low-pathogenicity avian influenza, caused by H7N1 type A influenza virus, affected the intensively-reared poultry population of Northeastern Italy [39]. Flocks, especially meat turkeys, were affected, with only a limited number of turkey breeder, chicken (breeders, broilers, and table egg layers), and guinea fowl flocks infected [39]. This outbreak eventually became virulent by mutation. Mannelli et al. said that turkey flocks were characterized by greater infection risk of high pathogenic influenza virus compared with other bird species such as layer hens, broilers, gamebirds, and waterfowl, even when located at distances more than 1.5 km from infected premises [40]. Mulatti et al. performed a spatial analysis of the 1999-2000 highly-pathogenic avian influenza H7N1 epidemic in northern Italy [41]. Mulatti et al. reported that the results highlighted the role of proximity in the spread of avian influenza virus and, when considering the Temporal Risk Window, indicated the possible direction of virus spread [41]. Di Trani et al. studied the molecular characterization of low pathogenicity H7N3 avian influenza viruses isolated in Italy [42]. According to this work, phylogenetic analyses of HA, PB2, and M genes showed that H7N3 and H7N1 viruses were closely related [42]. In addition, sequence analysis revealed a 23 amino acid deletion in the stalk of the neuraminidase of H7N3 viruses and a unique deletion of amino acid glycine in position 17 in the NP gene of H7N1 virus [42].

C. H7N2

H7N2 also ranks as an important avian influenza and is a cause of many previous avian influenza outbreaks among avian species. There are many reports from the United States.

Recently, an avian influenza outbreak occurred in meat-type chickens in central Pennsylvania from December 2001 to January 2002 [43]. According to this outbreak, two broiler breeder flocks were initially infected almost simultaneously in early December and avian influenza virus, H7N2 subtype, was isolated [43]. Clinical signs and lesions in broilers, when present, were compatible with multicausal respiratory disease [44]. With the exception of one broiler flock that was processed, birds from all of the virus positive flocks were euthanatized in-house within 11 days of the original case submission date [44]. A similar outbreak occurred from December of 1996 through April of 1998. This outbreak resulted in infection of 2,623,116 commercial birds on 25 premises encompassing 47 flocks [45]. The outbreak was believed to have originated from two separate introductions into commercial layer flocks from premises and by individuals dealing in sales of live fowl in the metropolitan New York and New Jersey live-bird markets [45]. Mixed fowl sold included ducks, geese, guinea hens, quail, partridges, and a variety of chickens grown on hundreds of small avian farms [45]. In 2004, the H7N2 subtype of avian influenza virus (AIV) field isolate (H7N2/chicken/PA/3779-2/97), which caused the 1997-98 AIV outbreak in Pennsylvania, was evaluated for its infectivity, length of infection, and immune response in specific-pathogen-free chickens by Lu and Castro [46]. Lu and Castro reported that H7N2 subtype of AIV induced a measurable immune response in all birds within 2 weeks after virus exposure and antibody titers were associated with avian influenza infectious doses and age of exposure of birds [46]. The latest outbreak of low-pathogenicity H7N2 avian influenza virus (AIV) in the Shenandoah Valley of Virginia that took place during the spring and summer of 2002 affected 197 farms and resulted in the destruction of over 4.7 million birds [47]. The virus primarily affected turkey flocks, causing respiratory distress and decreased egg production [48]. The successful eradication of this outbreak was the result of the efforts of a highly effective task force of industry, state, and federal personnel [47]. Tumpey et al. demonstrated the potential benefit of using an antigenically related 1997 H7N2 virus as a vaccine candidate for protection in poultry against a H7N2 virus isolate from 2002 [48]. McQuiston et al. performed another interesting study to identify risk factors associated with the spread of avian influenza virus among commercial poultry farms in western Virginia during an outbreak in 2002 [49]. According to this study, McQuiston et al. reported that an important factor contributing to rapid early spread of avian influenza virus infection among commercial poultry farms during this outbreak was disposal of dead birds via rendering off-farm [49]. McQuiston et al. concluded that poultry farmers should consider carcass disposal techniques that do not require off-farm movement, such as burial, composting, or incineration [49].

D. H7N3

H7N3 is another important avian influenza. H7N3 is a cause of many previous avian influenza outbreaks among avian species. In spring 2004, an outbreak of highly pathogenic avian influenza, subtype H7N3, occurred in the Fraser Valley of British Columbia, Canada [50]. Skowronski et al. said that compliance with recommended protective measures, especially goggles, was incomplete during the outbreak [51]. They noted that multiple back-up precautions, including oseltamivir prophylaxis, might prevent human infections and should be readily accessible and consistently used by those involved in the control of future outbreaks of avian influenza in poultry [51]. According to this outbreak, the British Columbia poultry industry, in collaboration with the British Columbia Ministry of Agriculture and Lands, developed an Enhanced Biosecurity Initiative that included the identification of mandatory on-farm biosecurity standards for commercial producers, an educational biosecurity self-assessment guide, and provisions for a producer self-quarantine to be enacted upon the first suspicion of disease [50].

E. H7N4

H7N4 is another important avian influenza is H7N4, a cause of many previous avian influenza outbreaks among avian species. In November of 1997, an outbreak of highly pathogenic avian influenza occurred near the town of Tamworth, in northern New South Wales, Australia [52]. There was no report on human infection from H7N4.

F. H7N7

H7N7 is another important avian influenza. H7N7 is a cause of many previous avian influenza outbreaks among avian species. The well-known outbreaks were documented in Germany and in the Netherlands. Rohm et al. said that the hemagglutinin genes from four avian H7N7 influenza A isolates, from a single outbreak, were shown to possess different cleavage sites that contained varying numbers of basic amino acid residues (KKKKR, KRKKR, KKRKKR, KKKKKKR) [53]. Rohm said that the degree of pathogenicity in vivo was not exclusively determined by the degree of hemagglutinin cleavability [53]. Elbers et al. said that the presence of apathy, decreased growth performance, reduction of normal vocalization, swollen sinuses, yawning, huddling, mucosal production from the beak, or lying down with an extended neck in infected turkey flocks appeared to be overall the most sensitive indicators to detect an outbreak, matching a sensitivity of 100% with a specificity of 79% [54].

G. H9N8

H9N8 is a new important avian influenza. Recently, an H5N8 outbreak occurred in South Korea. Low pathogenic avian influenza subtype H9N8 was diagnosed on a Korean native chicken farm in Gyeonggi province, South Korea, in late April 2004 [55]. This is the first report of an outbreak of low-pathogenic avian influenza in chickens caused by AIV subtype H9N8 [55].

H. H5N1

H5N1 is the cause of present epidemics in several regions of the world. H5N1 has become the new focus at present. Hundreds of human infected cases have been reported.

Pandemic of this infection is expected. H5N1 infection becomes a new emerging infectious disease under surveillance. More details on H5N1 infection are presented in other chapters of this book.

References

[1]   Kiselev OI, Sominina AA, Grinbaum EB. Influenza: current status and epidemiologic situation. Vestn Ross Akad Med Nauk. 1994;(9):3-7.

[2]   Hosrtmann DM. Clinical virology. *Am. J. Med.* 1965 May;38:738-50.

[3]   Skehel JJ, Wiley DC. Influenza viruses and cell membranes. *Am. J. Respir. Crit. Care Med.* 1995 Oct;152(4 Pt 2):S13-5.

[4]   Nayak DP, Hui EK, Barman S. Assembly and budding of influenza virus. *Virus Res.* 2004 Dec;106(2):147-65.

[5]   Schmitt AP, Lamb RA. Escaping from the cell: assembly and budding of negative-strand RNA viruses. *Curr. Top Microbiol. Immunol.* 2004;283:145-96.

[6]   Schulman JL. Influenza. *Postgrad Med.* 1971 Nov;50(5):171-5.

[7]   Webster RG, Laver WG. Antigenic variation in influenza virus. Biology and chemistry. *Prog. Med Virol.* 1971;13:271-338.

[8]   Moisa I. Recent acquisitions in the biology of influenza viruses. *Stud. Cercet Inframicrobiol.* 1971;22(2):143-70.

[9]   Maeda Y, Horimoto T, Kawaoka Y. Classification and genome structure of influenza virus. *Nippon Rinsho.* 2003 Nov;61(11):1886-91.

[10] Cheung TK, Poon LL. Biology of influenza a virus. *Ann. N Y Acad Sci.* 2007 Apr;1102:1-25.

[11] Nakajima K. Influenza virus genome structure and encoded proteins. *Nippon Rinsho.* 1997 Oct;55(10):2542-6.

[12] Scholtissek C. Molecular evolution of influenza viruses. *Virus Genes.* 1995;11(2-3):209-15.

[13] Moisa I. Theoretical considerations on the natural variability of influenza virus. *Stud. Cercet Inframicrobiol.* 1969;20(5):413-24.

[14] Fazekas de St Groth. Evolution and hierarchy of influenza viruses. *Arch. Environ. Health* 1970 Sep;21(3):293-303.

[15] Nakajima K, Nobusawa E, Nakajima S. Molecular evolution of influenza A virus. Uirusu. 1986 Dec;36(2):253-62.

[16] Ghendon YZ. Influenza virus RNA. *Acta Virol.* 1982 Jul;26(4):295-300.

[17] Ina Y, Gojobori T. Statistical analysis of nucleotide sequences of the hemagglutinin gene of human influenza A viruses. *Proc. Natl. Acad. Sci. U S A.* 1994 Aug 30;91(18):8388-92.

[19] Kanegae Y, Sugita S, Shortridge KF, Yoshioka Y, Nerome K. Origin and evolutionary pathways of the H1 hemagglutinin gene of avian, swine and human influenza viruses: cocirculation of two distinct lineages of swine virus. *Arch. Virol.* 1994;134(1-2):17-28.

[20] Nerome K, Kanegae Y, Yoshioka Y, Itamura S, Ishida M, Gojobori T, Oya A. Evolutionary pathways of N2 neuraminidases of swine and human influenza A viruses: origin of the neuraminidase genes of two reassortants (H1N2) isolated from pigs. *J. Gen Virol.* 1991 Mar;72 (Pt 3):693-8.

[21] Endo A, Pecoraro R, Sugita S, Nerome K. Evolutionary pattern of the H 3 haemagglutinin of equine influenza viruses: multiple evolutionary lineages and frozen replication. *Arch. Virol.* 1992;123(1-2):73-87.

[22] Daly JM, Lai AC, Binns MM, Chambers TM, Barrandeguy M, Mumford JA. Antigenic and genetic evolution of equine H3N8 influenza A viruses. *J. Gen. Virol.* 1996 Apr;77 (Pt 4):661-71.

[23] Lai AC, Chambers TM, Holland RE Jr, Morley PS, Haines DM, Townsend HG, Barrandeguy M. Diverged evolution of recent equine-2 influenza (H3N8) viruses in the Western Hemisphere. *Arch .Virol.* 2001;146(6):1063-74.

[24] Manuguerra JC, Zientara S, Sailleau C, Rousseaux C, Gicquel B, Rijks I, van der Werf S. Evidence for evolutionary stasis and genetic drift by genetic analysis of two equine influenza H3 viruses isolated in France. *Vet Microbiol.* 2000 May 22;74(1-2):59-70.

[25] Suarez DL. Evolution of avian influenza viruses. *Vet Microbiol.* 2000 May 22;74 (1-2):15-27.

[26] Kawaoka Y, Webster RG. Evolution of the A/Chicken/Pennsylvania/83 (H5N2) influenza virus. *Virology.* 1985 Oct 15;146(1):130-7.

[27] Cauthen AN, Swayne DE, Schultz-Cherry S, Perdue ML, Suarez DL. Continued circulation in China of highly pathogenic avian influenza viruses encoding the hemagglutinin gene associated with the 1997 H5N1 outbreak in poultry and humans. *J. Virol.* 2000 Jul;74(14):6592-9.

[28] Suarez DL, Senne DA, Banks J, Brown IH, Essen SC, Lee CW, Manvell RJ, Mathieu-Benson C, Moreno V, Pedersen JC, Panigrahy B, Rojas H, Spackman E, Alexander DJ. Recombination resulting in virulence shift in avian influenza outbreak, Chile. *Emerg. Infect Dis.* 2004 Apr;10(4):693-9.

[29] Spackman E, McCracken KG, Winker K, Swayne DE. H7N3 avian influenza virus found in a South American wild duck is related to the Chilean 2002 poultry outbreak, contains genes from equine and North American wild bird lineages, and is adapted to domestic turkeys. *J. Virol.* 2006 Aug;80(15):7760-4.

[30] Wood JM, Webster RG, Nettles VF. Host range of A/Chicken/Pennsylvania/83 (H5N2) influenza virus. *Avian Dis.* 1985 Jan-Mar;29(1):198-207.

[31] Kawaoka Y, Naeve CW, Webster RG. Is virulence of H5N2 influenza viruses in chickens associated with loss of carbohydrate from the hemagglutinin? *Virology.* 1984 Dec;139(2):303-16.

[32] Nettles VF, Wood JM, Webster RG. Wildlife surveillance associated with an outbreak of lethal H5N2 avian influenza in domestic poultry. *Avian Dis.* 1985 Jul-Sep;29(3): 733-41.

[33] Cappucci DT Jr, Johnson DC, Brugh M, Smith TM, Jackson CF, Pearson JE, Senne DA. Isolation of avian influenza virus (subtype H5N2) from chicken eggs during a natural outbreak. *Avian Dis*. 1985 Oct-Dec;29(4):1195-200.

[34] Wood JM, Kawaoka Y, Newberry LA, Bordwell E, Webster RG. Standardization of inactivated H5N2 influenza vaccine and efficacy against lethal A/Chicken/Pennsylvania /1370/83 infection. *Avian Dis*. 1985 Jul-Sep;29(3):867-72.

[35] Webster RG, Kawaoka Y, Bean WJ. Vaccination as a strategy to reduce the emergence of amantadine- and rimantadine-resistant strains of A/Chick/Pennsylvania/83 (H5N2) influenza virus. *J. Antimicrob. Chemother*. 1986 Oct;18 Suppl B:157-64.

[36] Donatelli I, Campitelli L, Di Trani L, Puzelli S, Selli L, Fioretti A, Alexander DJ, Tollis M, Krauss S, Webster RG. Characterization of H5N2 influenza viruses from Italian poultry. *J. Gen. Virol*. 2001 Mar;82(Pt 3):623-30.

[37] De Marco MA, Foni E, Campitelli L, Delogu M, Raffini E, Chiapponi C, Barigazzi G, Cordioli P, Di Trani L, Donatelli I. Influenza virus circulation in wild aquatic birds in Italy during H5N2 and H7N1 poultry epidemic periods (1998 to 2000). *Avian Pathol*. 2005 Dec;34(6):480-5.

[38] Capua I, Marangon S, dalla Pozza M, Terregino C, Cattoli G. Avian influenza in Italy 1997-2001. *Avian Dis*. 2003;47(3 Suppl):839-43.

[39] Mutinelli F, Capua I, Terregino C, Cattoli G. Clinical, gross, and microscopic findings in different avian species naturally infected during the H7N1 low- and high-pathogenicity avian influenza epidemics in Italy during 1999 and 2000. *Avian Dis*. 2003;47(3 Suppl):844-8.

[40] Mannelli A, Ferre N, Marangon S. Analysis of the 1999-2000 highly pathogenic avian influenza (H7N1) epidemic in the main poultry-production area in northern Italy. *Prev. Vet. Med*. 2006 Mar 16;73(4):273-85.

[41] Mulatti P, Kitron U, Mannelli A, Ferre N, Marangona S. Spatial analysis of the 1999-2000 highly pathogenic avian influenza (H7N1) epidemic in northern Italy. *Avian Dis*. 2007 Mar;51(1 Suppl):421-4.

[42] Di Trani L, Bedini B, Cordioli P, Muscillo M, Vignolo E, Moreno A, Tollis M. Molecular characterization of low pathogenicity H7N3 avian influenza viruses isolated in Italy. *Avian Dis*. 2004 Apr-Jun;48(2):376-83.

[43] Lu H, Dunn PA, Wallner-Pendleton EA, Henzler DJ, Kradel DC, Liu J, Shaw DP, Miller P. Investigation of H7N2 avian influenza outbreaks in two broiler breeder flocks in Pennsylvania, 2001-02. *Avian Dis*. 2004 Jan-Mar;48(1):26-33.

[44] Dunn PA, Wallner-Pendleton EA, Lu H, Shaw DP, Kradel D, Henzler DJ, Miller P, Key DW, Ruano M, Davison S. Summary of the 2001-02 Pennsylvania H7N2 low pathogenicity avian influenza outbreak in meat type chickens. *Avian Dis*. 2003;47(3 Suppl):812-6.

[45] Henzler DJ, Kradel DC, Davison S, Ziegler AF, Singletary D, DeBok P, Castro AE, Lu H, Eckroade R, Swayne D, Lagoda W, Schmucker B, Nesselrodt A. Epidemiology, production losses, and control measures associated with an outbreak of avian influenza subtype H7N2 in Pennsylvania (1996-98). *Avian Dis*. 2003;47(3 Suppl):1022-36.

[46] Lu H, Castro AE. Evaluation of the infectivity, length of infection, and immune response of a low-pathogenicity H7N2 avian influenza virus in specific-pathogen-free chickens. *Avian Dis.* 2004 Apr-Jun;48(2):263-70.

[47] Akey BL. Low-pathogenicity H7N2 avian influenza outbreak in Virgnia during 2002. *Avian Dis.* 2003;47(3 Suppl):1099-103.

[48] Tumpey TM, Kapczynski DR, Swayne DE. Comparative susceptibility of chickens and turkeys to avian influenza A H7N2 virus infection and protective efficacy of a commercial avian influenza H7N2 virus vaccine. *Avian Dis.* 2004 Jan-Mar;48(1):167-76.

[49] McQuiston JH, Garber LP, Porter-Spalding BA, Hahn JW, Pierson FW, Wainwright SH, Senne DA, Brignole TJ, Akey BL, Holt TJ. Evaluation of risk factors for the spread of low pathogenicity H7N2 avian influenza virus among commercial poultry farms. *J. Am. Vet. Med. Assoc.* 2005 Mar 1;226(5):767-72.

[50] Bowes VA. After the outbreak: how the British Columbia commercial poultry industry recovered after H7N3 HPAI. *Avian Dis.* 2007 Mar;51(1 Suppl):313-6.

[51] Skowronski DM, Li Y, Tweed SA, Tam TW, Petric M, David ST, Marra F, Bastien N, Lee SW, Krajden M, Brunham RC. Protective measures and human antibody response during an avian influenza H7N3 outbreak in poultry in British Columbia, Canada. *CMAJ.* 2007 Jan 2;176(1):47-53.

[52] Selleck PW, Arzey G, Kirkland PD, Reece RL, Gould AR, Daniels PW, Westbury HA. An outbreak of highly pathogenic avian influenza in Australia in 1997 caused by an H7N4 virus. *Avian Dis.* 2003;47(3 Suppl):806-11.

[53] Rohm C, Suss J, Pohle V, Webster RG. Different hemagglutinin cleavage site variants of H7N7 in an influenza outbreak in chickens in Leipzig, Germany. *Virology.* 1996 Apr 1;218(1):253-7.

[54] Elbers AR, Koch G, Bouma A. Performance of clinical signs in poultry for the detection of outbreaks during the avian influenza A (H7N7) epidemic in The Netherlands in 2003. *Avian Pathol.* 2005 Jun;34(3):181-7.

[55] Kwon YK, Lee YJ, Choi JG, Lee EK, Jeon WJ, Jeong OM, Kim MC, Joh SJ, Kwon JH, Kim JH. An outbreak of avian influenza subtype H9N8 among chickens in South Korea. *Avian Pathol.* 2006 Dec;35(6):443-7.

Chapter 1

The Emergence of Bird Flu, a Global Problem

History of Previous Influenza Pandemics

In history, there have been three will-documented previous influenza pandemics.

1. Spanish Flu [1 – 8]

Spanish flu is a pandemic caused by the H1N1 influenza virus. This pandemic occurred during the past two centuries. The pandemic started from Spain in Europe and spread around the world. This pandemic caused about 20-40 million deaths of the global population [9]. According to the study by Taubenberger et al., the H1N1 virus still crenellates into the present environment. RNA from a victim of the 1918 pandemic was isolated from a formalin-fixed, paraffin-embedded, lung tissue sample [10]. According to this work, nine fragments of viral RNA were sequenced from the coding regions of hemagglutinin, neuraminidase, nucleoprotein, matrix protein 1, and matrix protein 2 and the sequences were consistent with a novel H1N1 influenza A virus that belonged to the subgroup of strains that infect humans and swine, not the avian subgroup [10]. Reid et al. said that phylogenetic analyses suggested that the 1918 virus HA gene, although more closely related to avian strains than any other mammalian sequence, was mammalian and might have been adapting in humans before 1918 [11]. Reid et al. concluded that the hemagglutinin and nucleoprotein genome segments in particular were unlikely to have come directly from an avian source that is similar to those that are currently being sequenced [12].

Tumpey et al. reported that the 1918 pandemic virus had the ability to replicate in the absence of trypsin, caused death in mice and embryonated chicken eggs, and displayed a high-growth phenotype in human bronchial epithelial cells [13]. They also noted that the coordinated expression of the 1918 virus genes most certainly conferred the unique high-virulence phenotype observed with this pandemic virus [13]. Gibbs et al. said that reanalysis indicated that the hemagglutinin gene, a key virulence determinant, originated by recombination [14]. Gibbs et al. noted that the globular domain of the 1918 hemagglutinin protein was encoded by a part of a gene derived from swine-lineage influenza, whereas the stalk was encoded by parts derived from human-lineage influenza [14]. Gibbs et al. also reported that phylogenetic analyses showed that this recombination, which probably changed the virulence of the virus, occurred at the start of, or immediately before, the pandemic and thus might have triggered it [14]. However, Brownlee and Fodor could specify the extent of divergence of antigenic sites of the hemagglutinin during the antigenic drift of the virus between 1918 and 1934 based on the sequence of the haemagglutinin of the 1918 Spanish influenza [15]. This divergence was much more extensive than the divergence in predicted antigenic sites between the 1918 Spanish influenza and an avian H1 subtype consensus sequence [15]. These results support the hypothesis that the human 1918 pandemic originated from an avian virus of the H1 subtype that crossed the species barrier from birds to humans and adapted to humans, presumably by mutation and reassortment, shortly before 1918 [15]. Recently, Kobasa et al. reported that hemagglutinin of the 1918 virus conferred enhanced pathogenicity in mice to recent human viruses that were otherwise non-pathogenic in this host [16]. Kobasa et al. also reported that these highly virulent recombinant viruses expressing the 1918 viral hemagglutinin could have infected the entire lung and induced high levels of macrophage-derived chemokines and cytokines, which resulted in infiltration of inflammatory cells and severe hemorrhage [16].

2. Asian Flu [17 - 18]

Asian flu is a pandemic caused by the H2N2 influenza virus. This pandemic occurred during the past half century. H2N2 influenza A viruses caused the Asian pandemic of 1957 and then disappeared from the human population 10 years later [19]. This pandemic originated in China and spread to many countries. This pandemic caused about 2 million deaths among the Asian population. Schafer et al. determined the antigenicity of H2 hemagglutinins from representative human and avian H2 viruses and then analyzed the nucleotide and amino acid sequences to determine their evolutionary characteristics in different hosts [19]. Schafer et al. noted that antigenically conserved counterparts of the human Asian pandemic strain of 1957 continued to circulate in the avian reservoir and were coming into closer proximity to susceptible human populations [19]. Nerome et al. said that antigenic analysis by different antisera against H2N2 viruses and monoclonal antibodies to both the hemagglutinin and neuraminidase antigens showed that an avian isolate, A/duck/München/9/79, contained hemagglutinin and neuraminidase subunits closely related to those of the early human H2N2 viruses which had been prevalent in 1957 [20]. Nerome et al. also indicated that the oligonucleotide mapping showed that different H2N2 influenza virus variants had co-circulated in humans in 1957 [20].

3. Hong Kong Flu [21 – 30]

The Hong Kong flu is the most recent pandemic of influenza. This pandemic occurred during the past forty years. This pandemic started in Hong Kong and spread to many nearby countries. This pandemic has caused about 750,000 deaths among the Asian population. The main cause of death is pneumonia [31 – 33] In 2003, Ha et al. determined the structure of the HA of an avian influenza virus, A/duck/Ukraine/63, a member of the same antigenic subtype, H3, as the virus that caused the 1968 Hong Kong influenza pandemic, and a possible progenitor of the pandemic virus [34]. Ha et al. found that structurally significant differences between the avian and the human hemagglutinins were restricted to the receptor-binding site particularly the substitutions Q226L and G228S that caused the site to open and residues within it to rearrange, including the conserved residues Y98, W153, and H183 [34]. Skehel et al. reported that addition of the new oligosaccharide side chain was required for Hong Kong influenza epidemic A/England/878/69, which contained a hemagglutinin glycosylated at residue 63, to prevent reaction with the monoclonal antibody [35].

Emergence of H1N1 Bird Flu Epidemic [36 - 50]

Emergence of the H1N1 bird flu started during the past 10 years. The brief context of the epidemic is listed in Table 1.

Table 1. Brief consequence of H1N1 epidemic

Period	Details
1997	The first human H5N1 infection was reported. This incidence occurred in Hong Kong. There were 18 cases of human H5N1 infections in this epidemic. Of 18 infected cases, 6 died. The history taking and disease tracing showed that all infected cases had history of contact to avians. This is the first episode of H5N1 infection in a human.
2003	In December 2003, a big epidemic of H5N1 virus in domestic avians occurred in many counties including Thailand, Korea, Japan and Vietnam. Destroying of suspected avians was performed.
January	The first two cases of human H5N1 infection in Thailand were reported. These two cases were predicative patients with history of closed contact with the domestic chickens in their houses. This is the starting point of concern regarding human infection in Thailand.
March	Thailand successfully controlled the H5N1 epidemic, 12 infected cases. A number of chickens were destroyed in the disease control process.
August	The H5N1 epidemic occurred in Vietminh. There were repeats of human H5N1 infection and deaths.
September	Thailand reported a new episode of H5N1 attack. There were 17 infected cases with 12 fatal cases. Bird flu in a tiger occurred. This was a new finding and drew the interest of scientists all over the world. The epidemic occurred at a Tiber tanning farm named "Suan Suer Sriracha" near a famous sea resort, Pattaya, in Thailand.
December	Repeated human epidemics occurred in Vietnam and there were additional human infections in many countries including Thailand, Vietnam, Cambodia,

Table 1. (Continued)

Period	Details
	Indonesia and China following this episode.
2004 February	The first human H5N1 infected case was reported in Cambodia. A total of four were 4 infected, and all died.
July	The first human H5N1 infected case was reported in Indonesia. In the same period, an epidemic in avians occurred in Russia.
September	There were epidemics of H5N1 in avians in Turkey and Romania. Also, there were additional human H5M1 infected cases in Indonesia.
October	The third epidemic occurred in Thailand. There were five human infected cases. Human H5N1 infected cases were reported in China. There were five human infected cases. Additionally, an epidemic in world birds occurred in Croatia.

A. Human H5N1 Infection in Thailand [51 – 55]

As previously mentioned, human H5N1 cases have been reported since the first H5N1 episode in Thailand in 2004. The first two human cases in Thailand were children living in the Kanchanaburi and Suphanburi provinces in Central Regions of Thailand. These two children had a history of close contact with their families' domestic childrens. They played and lived with infected chickens. At first, these two children were diagnosed with simple bird flu. Their symptoms progressed and, finally, they died. In the first episode in 2004, there was a total of 10 human H5N1 cases and 8 died. In the second episode, there were an additional five human infected cases, and four died. In the third and last episode in 2005, five human cases could be detected. However, the fatality decreased; only two people died. This implies a better management program and use of antiviral drugs.

Table 2. Summary of human H5N1 infection and mortality in Thailand

Penned	Number*	
	Infection	death
Dec 03 – Mar 04	12	8
Jul 04 – Oct 04	5	4
Dec 04 – Oct 05	5	2

All but one confirmed infected cases according to the WHO definition: positive influenza A H5N1 culture and/or positive H5 by RT-PCR method and/a positive 4-fold rising of H5-specific antibody.

B. Human H5N1 Infection in Vietnam [52, 56]

Emerging H5N1 infection in Vietnam occurred during the same period as that in Thailand.

A high fatality was reported. Vietnam is believed to be the source of the present epidemic of H5N1 infection. More details on human H5N1 infection in Vietnam will be discussed in another section of this book.

Factors Contributing to the Emergence of Bird Flu

Similar to general disorders in medicine, two main factors contributing to the emergence of bird flu are inherited and non-inherited factors.

1. Inherited Factors

Host Susceptibility

Truly, the inherited factor has been extensively studied for its role in response to many illnesses, especially for response to contagious illnesses. The effect of host genetics on the susceptibility to influenza virus has been studied for years. According to the study of Mackenzy et al., the effect of two host genetic factors on the outcome of influenza A infections has been examined: ABO blood groups and HL-A antigens [57]. According to this study, no difference was observed in the ability of subjects of different blood groups to seroconvert after receiving two doses of live attenuated influenza A vaccine, but a significantly higher proportion of blood group A vaccines seroconverted after receiving their first dose of vaccine [57]. In addition, the association between HL-A type BW16 and resistance to infection with influenza could not be confirmed [57]. Mackenzie and Fimmel performed a similar study. According to their study, higher geometric mean HI antibody titres were observed in blood group O subjects after the administration of killed subunit vaccine [58]. The results described in this report supported the contention that genetic factors linked to ABO blood groups may play a role in susceptibility to infection with influenza A virus, but that any association must be indirect [58]. Gelder et al. concluded that polymorphisms in HLA class II molecules appeared to modulate antibody responses to influenza vaccination [59]. Lambkin et al. recently conducted a small study to investigate whether there were any association between HLA class II molecules and nonresponsiveness to influenza virus vaccination [60]. This work revealed that the HLA-DRB1*0701 allele was over-represented among persons who fail to mount a neutralizing antibody response [60]. This preliminary finding is important because it potentially identifies a group who may not be protected by current vaccination strategies [60]. It seems that the studies of host genetic susceptibility for bird flu are very limited. Further research to discover new knowledge on this area are suggested.

Susceptibility of Pathogens

Besides host susceptibility, the susceptibility of a pathogen to an anti-pathogenic agent is also extensively investigated. Drug-resistant influenza virus is reported [61 - 62]. At present, it is accepted that the H5N1 strains are resistant to amantadine and rimantadine but are susceptible to neuraminidase inhibitors, which can be used for treatment and prophylaxis [63]. More details on the drug resistance of bird flu virus can be seen in Chapter 9 on treatment of bird flu in this book.

Genetic Mutation and Recombination

Genetic mutation and recombination are believed to be the most important factor scontributing to the emerging and possible pandemic of bird flu in humans. Type A influenza viruses are classified in different sub-types depending of the nature of their surface glycoproteins: haemagglutinin and neuraminidase [64]. The nature of the genome and the mode of replication of influenza viruses account for the high variability of these two proteins which are responsible for the immunity to the virus [64]. Two kinds of minor antigenic variations, producing new strains within type A virus subtypes, have been discovered: antigenic drift, in which the amino acid sequences of the antigens are changed; and antigenic camouflage, in which the antigens are glycosylated [65]. Both kinds of variation are caused by mutations in the viral genome [65]. In contrast to infectious agents causing classical zoonoses, influenza viruses have to alter their genetic composition in order to change their host range [66]. The special, segmented structure of the viral RNA allows an exchange of genes between two different influenza viruses (reassortment) resulting in viruses with different combinations of genome segments and thereby creating new biological properties [66]. Day et al. recently developed a stochastic model for the evolutionary emergence of pandemic influenza [67]. Day et al. found that if evolutionary emergence of past pandemics had occurred primarily through viral reassortment in humans, then thousands of avian influenza virus infections in humans should have occurred each year for the past 250 years [67]. Day et al. also proposed that there was epidemiologically significant variation among avian influenza virus genotypes; therefore, then avian virus outbreaks stemming from repeated cross-species transmission events resulted in a greater likelihood of a pandemic strain evolving than those caused by low-level transmission between humans [67].

2. Non-Inherited Factor

Poverty

Poverty creates a lack of opportunity for maintaining good health; and brings with it many disorders, especially tropical infections. Low income is a main barrier to access to good health services [68]. During the 1918-1919 outbreak of influenza in the British Caribbean, the heaviest mortality rates were among the very poor [69]. In a recent study by Ompad et al. [70], economic and racial disparities in influenza vaccine access in times of adequate supply and the inability to distribute the vaccine due to the shortage were assessed. According to this work, few people were vaccinated: vaccination rates for adults in priority groups and non-priority groups were 21.0% and 3.5%, respectively [70]. The association between poverty and bird flu infection in humans has been confirmed [71 - 72]. Therefore, development based on economic growth to conquer poverty in tropical countries is necessary and becomes a political strategy for all developing countries. The process of urbanization can be described as one of the greater global environmental changes directly affecting human health and affected populations, especially in developing countries where urban growth like an express train had been accompanied by massive urban poverty.

Poor Hygiene

As previously mentioned, poor hygiene can be the result of poverty. The population tropical places, especially marginal groups, in generally receives few sanitary services. For influenza, poor hygiene is an important factor contributing to contracting the disease. Tangkanakul et al. recently studied an outbreak of Influenza A virus in a hilltribe village of Mae Hong Son Province in Thailand [73]. Tangkanakul et al. found that predisposing factors of the village that might have influenced the outbreak included crowded living quarters, cold and moist weather, poor personal hygiene and improper sanitation [73]. Angelava and Angelava said that humans became infected by eating infected birds, by poor hygiene procedures when cooking infected birds, or by close contact with infected poultry [74]. Therefore, sanitation is at the heart of preventive control of bird flu.

Environmental Temperature and Humidity

Similar to other tropical illnesses, the environmental temperature, which is generally hot in the tropics, aids the transmission of influenza. There are many investigations into the effect of temperature on influenza. For bird flu, environmental temperature has important effect on the viral transmission. Brown et al. reported that 1) H5 and H7 avian influenza viruses could persist for extended periods of time in water, with a duration of infectivity comparable to influenza viruses of other subtypes; 2) the persistence of H5 and H7 influenza viruses was inversely proportional to temperature and salinity of water; and 3) a significant interaction exists between the effects of temperature and salinity on the persistence of influenza virus, with the effect of salinity more prominent at lower temperatures [75]. Chumpolbanchorn et al. recently studied the effect of temperature on infectivity of avian influenza virus (H5N1, Thai field strain) in chicken fecal manure [76]. They found that at 25 degrees C the virus lost its infectivity within 24 hours and at 40 degrees C within 15 minutes [76]. Shortridge et al. reported that transmission experiments in chickens revealed that the H5N1 viruses were spread by fecal-oral transmission rather than by aerosol, and that the viruses were inactivated by drying feces at ambient temperature; however, infectivity was maintained for at least 4 days in wet feces at 25 degrees C [77].

Pollution

Exposure to environmental contamination remains a main source of health risk throughout the world, although risks are generally higher in developing countries. For bird flu, among the many risk factors that may be important are alterations in host immunity, malnutrition, prior or coincident infections with other microorganisms, inhaled pollutants, and lack of access to medical care [78]. At present, change in climate is also an important factor in the discussion on world health. Urashima et al. suggested that most of the oscillation in the number of influenza cases might be explained using a seasonal model that can simulate the impact of global warming [79]. Urashima et al. reported that if the number of days with both maximum temperature greater than or equal to 10 degress C and relative humidity less than 60% increased by one per week, the number of influenza cases was simulated to decrease by approximately half [79].

Public Health Significance of Bird Flu

Bird flu infection is a global concern. It is classified as a new emerging disease. Basically, a great global environmental change occurred within this century due to recently growing industrialization. Transportation has become faster than previous years. There are many incursions of cities into the forests bringing wild pathogens back into the cities. The world population has increased and become poor proportionate to the limited area. Farming systems are not well controlled in many countries. In addition, the global warming effect has affected many regions all around the world. These factors help generate many new emerging infectious diseases. Bird flu infection in humans is also believed to be based on these facts. Further research is required to better define conditions under which the influenza virus may transmit via the airborne route [80]. More international funding from both human and animal health agencies for diagnosis or detection and control of bird flu is needed [81]. Finally, additional funding for research is needed to understand why and how these bird flu viruses infect humans and what pandemic risks they pose [81].

References

[1]   Webster RG. 1918 Spanish influenza: the secrets remain elusive. *Proc. Natl. Acad. Sci. U S A*. 1999 Feb 16;96(4):1164-6.

[2]   Shortridge KF. The 1918 'Spanish' flu: pearls from swine? *Nat. Med.* 1999 Apr;5(4):384-5.

[3]   Pennisi E. First genes isolated from the deadly 1918 flu virus. *Science.* 1997 Mar 21;275(5307):1739.

[4]   Kaiser J. Virology. Resurrected influenza virus yields secrets of deadly 1918 pandemic. *Science.* 2005 Oct 7;310(5745):28-9.

[5]   Shortridge KF. The 1918 'Spanish' flu: pearls from swine? *Nat. Med.* 1999 Apr;5(4):384-5.

[6]   Taubenberger JK, Reid AH, Fanning TG. The 1918 influenza virus: A killer comes into view. *Virology.* 2000 Sep 1;274(2):241-5.

[7]   Enserink M. Influenza. What came before 1918? Archaeovirologist offers a first glimpse. *Science.* 2006 Jun 23;312(5781):1725.

[8]   Study of 1918 influenza pandemic virus provides information on origin and virulence mechanisms. *Euro Surveill.* 2005 Oct 20;10(10):E051020.1.

[9]   Reid AH, Taubenberger JK, Fanning TG. The 1918 Spanish influenza: integrating history and biology. *Microbes Infect.* 2001 Jan;3(1):81-7.

[10] Taubenberger JK, Reid AH, Krafft AE, Bijwaard KE, Fanning TG. Initial genetic characterization of the 1918 "Spanish" influenza virus. *Science.* 1997 Mar 21;275(5307):1793-6.

[11] Reid AH, Fanning TG, Hultin JV, Taubenberger JK. Origin and evolution of the 1918 "Spanish" influenza virus hemagglutinin gene. *Proc. Natl. Acad. Sci. U S A.* 1999 Feb 16;96(4):1651-6.

[12] Reid AH, Taubenberger JK, Fanning TG. Evidence of an absence: the genetic origins of the 1918 pandemic influenza virus. *Nat. Rev. Microbiol.* 2004 Nov;2(11):909-14.

[13] Tumpey TM, Basler CF, Aguilar PV, Zeng H, Solorzano A, Swayne DE, Cox NJ, Katz JM, Taubenberger JK, Palese P, Garcia-Sastre A. Characterization of the reconstructed 1918 Spanish influenza pandemic virus. *Science.* 2005 Oct 7;310(5745):77-80.

[14] Brownlee GG, Fodor E. The predicted antigenicity of the haemagglutinin of the 1918 Spanish influenza pandemic suggests an avian origin. *Philos. Trans. R Soc. Lond B. Biol. Sci.* 2001 Dec 29;356(1416):1871-6.

[15] Gibbs MJ, Armstrong JS, Gibbs AJ. Recombination in the hemagglutinin gene of the 1918 "Spanish flu". *Science.* 2001 Sep 7;293(5536):1842-5.

[16] Kobasa D, Takada A, Shinya K, Hatta M, Halfmann P, Theriault S, Suzuki H, Nishimura H, Mitamura K, Sugaya N, Usui T, Murata T, Maeda Y, Watanabe S, Suresh M, Suzuki T, Suzuki Y, Feldmann H, Kawaoka Y. Enhanced virulence of influenza A viruses with the haemagglutinin of the 1918 pandemic virus. *Nature.* 2004 Oct 7;431(7009):703-7.

[17] Levine R. A cure for the Asian flu. *Biosecur. Bioterror.* 2006;4(3):228-30.

[18] Kilbourne ED. Influenza pandemics: past, present and future. *J. Formos. Med. Assoc.* 2006 Jan;105(1):1-6.

[19] Schafer JR, Kawaoka Y, Bean WJ, Suss J, Senne D, Webster RG. Origin of the pandemic 1957 H2 influenza A virus and the persistence of its possible progenitors in the avian reservoir. *Virology.* 1993 Jun;194(2):781-8.

[20] Nerome K, Yoshioka Y, Torres CA, Oya A, Bachmann P, Ottis K, Webster RG. Persistence of Q strain of H2N2 influenza virus in avian species: antigenic, biological and genetic analysis of avian and human H2N2 viruses. *Arch. Virol.* 1984;81(3-4):239-50.

[21] Cockburn WC, Delon PJ, Ferreira W. Origin and progress of the 1968-69 Hong Kong influenza epidemic. *Bull. World Health Organ.* 1969;41(3):345-8.

[22] Buescher EL, Smith TJ, Zachary IH. Experience with Hong Kong influenza in tropical areas. *Bull. World Health Organ.* 1969;41(3):387-91.

[23] Chang WK. National influenza experience in Hong Kong, 1968. *Bull. World Health Organ.* 1969;41(3):349-51.

[24] White PC Jr. A2-Hong Kong-68. *Va. Med. Mon.* (1918). 1968 Oct;95(10):595-6.

[25] Hrabar A, Ugrcic I. A-2 Hong Kong influenza epidemic in Croatia in 1969-70. *Lijec Vjesn.* 1972 Mar;94(3):125-31.

[26] Kundin WD. Hong Kong influenza. Serological, immunochemical and epidemiologic studies. *Taiwan Yi Xue Hui Za Zhi.* 1969 Nov 28;68(11):568-9.

[27] Davis LE, Caldwell GG, Lynch RE, Bailey RE, Chin TD. Hong Kong influenza: the epidemiologic features of a high school family study analyzed and compared with a

similar study during the 1957 Asian influenza epidemic. *Am. J. Epidemiol.* 1970 Oct;92(4):240-7.

[28] Influenza: the Hong Kong virus. WHO Chron. 1968 Dec;22(12):528-9.

[29] Vastag B. Hong Kong flu still poses pandemic threat. *JAMA.* 2002 Nov 20;288(19):2391-5.

[30] Hong Kong influenza: the coming winter. *Med. J. Aust.* 1970 Feb 21;1(8):393-4.

[31] Bisno AL, Griffin JP, Van Epps KA, Niell HB, Rytel MW. Pneumonia and Hong Kong influenza: a prospective study of the 1968-1969 epidemic. *Am. J. Med. Sci.* 1971 May;261(5):251-63.

[32] Schwarzmann SW, Adler JL, Sullivan RJ Jr, Marine WM. Bacterial pneumonia during the Hong Kong influenza epidemic of 1968-1969. *Arch. Intern. Med.* 1971 Jun;127(6):1037-41.

[33] Burk RF, Schaffner W, Koenig MG. Severe influenza virus pneumonia in the pandemic of 1968-1969. *Arch. Intern. Med.* 1971 Jun;127(6):1122-8.

[34] Ha Y, Stevens DJ, Skehel JJ, Wiley DC. X-ray structure of the hemagglutinin of a potential H3 avian progenitor of the 1968 Hong Kong pandemic influenza virus. *Virology.* 2003 May 10;309(2):209-18.

[35] Skehel JJ, Stevens DJ, Daniels RS, Douglas AR, Knossow M, Wilson IA, Wiley DC. A carbohydrate side chain on hemagglutinins of Hong Kong influenza viruses inhibits recognition by a monoclonal antibody. *Proc. Natl. Acad. Sci. U S A.* 1984 Mar;81(6):1779-83.

[36] Allen PJ. The world awaits the next pandemic: will it be H5N1, the 'bird flu'? *J. Child Health Care.* 2006 Sep;10(3):178-87.

[37] Wiwanitkit V. A typical bird flu infection, caused by the H5N1 virus, is a new emerging infectious disease. *J. Trauma.* 2006 Sep;61(3):768-9.

[38] Allen PJ. Avian influenza pandemic: not if, but when. *Pediatr. Nurs.* 2006 Jan-Feb;32(1):76-81.

[39] Davies K, Higginson R. The continuing threat of avian influenza. *Br. J. Nurs.* 2006 Apr 27-May 10;15(8):418.

[40] Barlow BG. The potential for a pandemic? What the renal professional and patient need to know about avian flu. *Nephrol. News Issues.* 2006 Aug;20(9):42-6.

[41] Clemison D. Preparing for an influenza pandemic. *Community Pract.* 2007 Jan;80(1):10-2.

[42] Rivera SJ. Avian influenza (H5N1)--the next pandemic? *Imprint.* 2006 Apr-May;53(3):56, 58, 62.

[43] Weber CJ. Update on preparing for the next influenza pandemic. *Dermatol. Nurs.* 2006 Aug;18(4):362-6.

[44] Weber CJ. Update on preparing for the next influenza pandemic. *Urol. Nurs.* 2006 Apr;26(2):145-8.

[45] McConnell J. The Lancet forum on preparing for pandemic influenza. *Lancet Infect. Dis.* 2006 Jul;6(7):390-2.

[46] Normile D. Avian influenza. WHO proposes plan to stop pandemic in its tracks. *Science.* 2006 Jan 20;311(5759):315-6.

[47] Nicoll A, Van-Tam J. World Health Organization finds no evidence that human influenza (H5N1) infections are spreading readily among humans in Vietnam. *Euro Surveill.* 2005 Jul 7;10(7):E050707.3.

[48] Sampathkumar P, Maki DG. Avian H5N1 influenza--are we inching closer to a global pandemic? *Mayo Clin. Proc.* 2005 Dec;80(12):1552-5.

[49] Vague-Rafart J. The threat of avian influenza human pandemic. *Med. Clin.* (Barc). 2006 Feb 11;126(5):183-8.

[50] Sheff B. Avian influenza: poised to launch a pandemic? *Nursing.* 2006 Jan;36(1):51-3.

[51] Tiensin T, Chaitaweesub P, Songserm T, Chaisingh A, Hoonsuwan W, Buranathai C, Parakamawongsa T, Premashthira S, Amonsin A, Gilbert M, Nielen M, Stegeman A. Highly pathogenic avian influenza H5N1, Thailand, 2004. *Emerg. Infect. Dis.* 2005 Nov;11(11):1664-72.

[52] Lipatov AC, Smirnov IuA, Kaverin NV, Webster RG. Evolution of avian influenza viruses H5N1 (1997-2004) in southern and south-eastern Asia. *Vopr. Virusol.* 2005 Jul-Aug;50(4):11-7.

[53] Tiensin T, Nielen M, Songserm T, Kalpravidh W, Chaitaweesub P, Amonsin A, Chotiprasatintara S, Chaisingh A, Damrongwatanapokin S, Wongkasemjit S, Antarasena C, Songkitti V, Chanachai K, Thanapongtham W, Stegeman JA.Geographic and temporal distribution of highly pathogenic avian influenza A virus (H5N1) in Thailand, 2004-2005: an overview. *Avian Dis.* 2007 Mar;51(1 Suppl):182-8.

[54] Songserm T, Jam-on R, Sae-Heng N, Meemak N, Hulse-Post DJ, Sturm-Ramirez KM, Webster RG. Domestic ducks and H5N1 influenza epidemic, Thailand. *Emerg. Infect. Dis.* 2006 Apr;12(4):575-81.

[55] Buranathai C, Amonsin A, Chaisigh A, Theamboonlers A, Pariyothorn N, Poovorawan Y. Surveillance activities and molecular analysis of H5N1 highly pathogenic avian influenza viruses from Thailand, 2004-2005. *Avian Dis.* 2007 Mar;51(1 Suppl):194-200.

[56] Avian influenza A(H5N1) in humans and poultry, Vietnam. *Wkly Epidemiol. Rec.* 2004 Jan 16;79(3):13-4.

[57] Mackenzie JS, Wetherall JD, Fimmel PJ, Hawkins BR, Dawkins RL. Host factors and susceptibility to influenza A infection: the effect of ABO blood groups and HL-A antigens. *Dev. Biol. Stand.* 1977 Jun 1-3;39:355-62.

[58] Mackenzie JS, Fimmel PJ. The effect of ABO blood groups on the incidence of epidemic influenza and on the response to live attenuated and detergent split influenza virus vaccines. *J. Hyg (Lond).* 1978 Feb;80(1):21-30.

[59] Gelder CM, Lambkin R, Hart KW, Fleming D, Williams OM, Bunce M, Welsh KI, Marshall SE, Oxford J. Associations between human leukocyte antigens and nonresponsiveness to influenza vaccine. *J. Infect. Dis.* 2002 Jan 1;185(1):114-7.

[60] Lambkin R, Novelli P, O7xford J, Gelder C. Human genetics and responses to influenza vaccination: clinical implications. *Am. J. Pharmacogenomics.* 2004;4(5):293-8.

[61] Saito R, Suzuki H. Antiviral resistance of influenza viruses. *Nippon Rinsho.* 2007 Feb 28;65 Suppl 2 Pt. 1:471-5.

[62] Tsuji K, Iwahashi J, Imamura Y, Yoshimoto S, Kajiwara J, Ishibashi T, Mori R, Yamada T, Toyoda T. Emergence of amantadine-resistant influenza A viruses. *Uirusu.* 2001 Dec;51(2):135-41.

[63] Trampuz A, Prabhu RM, Smith TF, Baddour LM. Avian influenza: a new pandemic threat? *Mayo Clin. Proc.* 2004 Apr;79(4):523-30.

[64] Meulemans G. Inter-species transmission of the influenza virus. *Bull. Mem. Acad. R. Med. Belg.* 1999;154(5-6):263-70

[65] Kendal AP. Epidemiologic implications of changes in the influenza virus genome. *Am. J. Med.* 1987 Jun 19;82(6A):4-14.

[66] Rott R. Influenza, a special form of zoonosis. Berl Munch Tierarztl Wochenschr. 1997 Jul-Aug;110(7-8):241-6.

[67] Day T, Andre JB, Park A. The evolutionary emergence of pandemic influenza. *Proc. Biol. Sci.* 2006 Dec 7;273(1604):2945-53.

[68] Bergner L, Yerby AS. Low income and barriers to use of health services. *N. Engl. J. Med.* 1968 Mar 7;278(10):541-6.

[69] Killingray D. The influenza pandemic of 1918-1919 in the British Caribbean. *Soc. Hist. Med.* 1994 Apr;7(1):59-87.

[70] Ompad DC, Galea S, Blaney S, Coady MH, Sisco S, Glidden K, Vlahov D. Access to influenza vaccine in East Harlem and the Bronx during a national vaccine shortage. *J. Community Health.* 2007 Jun;32(3):195-202.

[71] Cristalli A, Capua I. Practical problems in controlling H5N1 high pathogenicity avian influenza at village level in Vietnam and introduction of biosecurity measures. *Avian Dis.* 2007 Mar;51(1 Suppl):461-2.

[72] Ferguson N. Poverty, death, and a future influenza pandemic. *Lancet.* 2006 Dec 23;368(9554):2187-8.

[73] Tangkanakul W, Tharmaphornpilas P, Thawatsupha P, Laolukpong P, Lertmongkol J. An outbreak of Influenza A virus in a hilltribe village of Mae Hong Son Province Thailand, 1997. *J. Med. Assoc. Thai.* 2000 Sep;83(9):1005-10.

[74] Angelava NA, Angelava AV. Epidemiology, clinical picture, prevention and treatment of Avian influenza. *Georgian Med. News.* 2006 Feb;(131):69-76.

[75] Brown JD, Swayne DE, Cooper RJ, Burns RE, Stallknecht DE. Persistence of H5 and H7 avian influenza viruses in water. *Avian Dis.* 2007 Mar;51(1 Suppl):285-9.

[76] Chumpolbanchorn K, Suemanotham N, Siripara N, Puyati B, Chaichoune K. The effect of temperature and UV light on infectivity of avian influenza virus (H5N1, Thai field strain) in chicken fecal manure. *Southeast Asian J. Trop. Med. Public Health.* 2006 Jan;37(1):102-5.

[77] Shortridge KF, Zhou NN, Guan Y, Gao P, Ito T, Kawaoka Y, Kodihalli S, Krauss S, Markwell D, Murti KG, Norwood M, Senne D, Sims L, Takada A, Webster RG. Characterization of avian H5N1 influenza viruses from poultry in Hong Kong. *Virology.* 1998 Dec 20;252(2):331-42.

[78] Leigh MW, Carson JL, Denny FW Jr. Pathogenesis of respiratory infections due to influenza virus: implications for developing countries. *Rev. Infect. Dis.* 1991 May-Jun;13 Suppl 6:S501-8.

[79] Urashima M, Shindo N, Okabe N. A seasonal model to simulate influenza oscillation in Tokyo. *Jpn. J. Infect. Dis.* 2003 Apr;56(2):43-7.

[80] Brankston G, Gitterman L, Hirji Z, Lemieux C, Gardam M. Transmission of influenza A in human beings. *Lancet Infect. Dis.* 2007 Apr;7(4):257-65.

[81] Perdue ML, Swayne DE. Public health risk from avian influenza viruses. *Avian Dis.* 2005 Sep;49(3):317-27.

Chapter 2

Bird Flu in China and East Asia

East Asia a Site for New Emerging Infectious Diseases [1 – 4]

East Asia, the easternmost area of the Asian continent, has a very long history. Oriental tradition is generated from East Asia. Of interest, in recent decades, East Asia has become an area of concern as a site for new emerging infectious diseases. A well-known phenomenon is severe acute respiratory syndrome (SARS) [5 - 11], which originated in China. There are many factors that led East Asia to be a site of many new emerging infectious diseases. First, it can be accepted that East Asia still preserves its natural reservoirs. Many undiscovered pathogens exist in the natural sites of East Asia. In addition, there are many deep-rooted traditional practices in East Asia. Some of these oriental traditions might lead to susceptibility to new emerging infectious diseases. Well-known risky behavior includes traditional eating habits. Many local populations in East Asia eat wild animals that can act as reservoirs for infectious agents. Second, there are many people living in East Asia. China is the country with the highest population. Crowded populations in some cities can lead to health problems [12 - 13]. Of interest, most people in East Asia have low incomes which can lead to health neglect or lack of access to good health services. Poverty is detrimental to good health. Poverty can lead to high susceptibility to contact with pathogens [14]. Third, the change in economical systems in East Asia affects natural sites [15]. Rapid growth of cities due to industrialization invades forests and discovered pathogens in contact with humans. Uncontollable growth of the cities can specifically affect the health status of the people in the new cities [16 - 17]. With rapid urbanization, slums grow. Poor sanitation systems in impoverished communities is the root cause of the epidemic of new emerging infectious diseases. In addition, control of new disease in a large community is very difficult. In addition, the traditional eating style of the East Asian population should be a concern [18]. Pork and chicken are the main sources of meat for the local populations in East Asia. In the case of bird flu, this can be considered a high risk. Among the many chicken and pig farms in East Asia, some are small in-house farm epidemic. Chicken meat and egg are a concern as the future probable source of bird flu epidemic [19]. Pigs can serve as the host in which human and avian influenza viruses can be combined. If sense mutation occurs, it can be the root cause of a future possible pandemic of bird flu. Woo et al. said that in Chinese wet-markets, unique epicenters for transmission of potential viral pathogens, new genes might be acquired or existing genes modified through various mechanisms such as genetic reassortment, recombination and mutation [20]. Woo et al. said that the wet-markets, at closer proximity to humans, with high viral burden or strains of higher transmission efficiency, facilitated transmission of the viruses to humans [20].

Bird Flu in Hong Kong

Hong Kong flu is a well-known influenza infection in the history [21 – 30]. Hong Kong was one of the first countries attacked by H5N1 infection.

The spread of highly pathogenic avian influenza A virus, subtype H5N1, in chicken farms during the first quarter of 2002 in Hong Kong was reported. According to the study of Kung et al., the risk for influenza A H5N1 infection was assessed by using adjusted odds ratios based on multivariate logistic regression analysis [31]. According to this work, retail marketing of live poultry was implicated as the main source of exposure to infection on chicken farms in Hong Kong during this period [31]. Kung et al. mentioned that infection control measures should be reviewed and upgraded as necessary to reduce the spread of influenza A H5N1 related to live poultry markets, which were commonplace across Asia [31]. Shortridge et al. said that each of the H5N1 viruses from Hong Kong poultry markets that were tested were lethal in chickens, possessed polybasic amino acids at the carboxy-terminus of HA1, and by definition were highly pathogenic in poultry [32]. Since the outbreak in humans of an H5N1 avian influenza virus in Hong Kong in 1997, poultry entering the live-bird markets of Hong Kong have been closely monitored for infection with avian influenza [33]. Cauthen reported that at least one of the avian influenza virus genes encoded by the 1997 H5N1 Hong Kong viruses continued to circulate in mainland China and that this gene was important for pathogenesis in chickens but is not the sole determinant of pathogenicity in mice [33]. Cauthen et al. noted that there was evidence that H9N2 viruses, which have internal genes in common with the 1997 H5N1 Hong Kong isolates, were still circulating in Hong Kong and China as well, providing a heterogeneous gene pool for viral reassortment [33]. Outbreaks of highly pathogenic H5N1 avian influenza also occurred in Hong Kong in chickens and other gallinaceous poultry in 2001, twice in 2002 and 2003 [34].

Infection in local chicken farms was preceded by the detection of virus in multiple retail markets and the main poultry wholesale market [35]. The first case of this disease on a local farm was detected on February 1, 2002. By February 9, 2002, 15 farms were infected, and by late March a total of 22 infected farms had been identified [35]. Control of this disease has been performed through a combination of quarantine, tightening of biosecurity measures, and depopulation of infected and contact farms [35]. About 950,000 birds have been destroyed [35]. Vaccination using a killed H5 vaccine was introduced in April 2002 to farms in one zone where infection has persisted [35]. Ellis reported an investigation of outbreaks of highly pathogenic H5N1 avian influenza in waterfowl and wild birds in Hong Kong in late 2002 [34]. Ellis et al. reported that the first waterfowl outbreak was controlled by immediate strict quarantine and depopulation one week before the second outbreak commenced [34]. Ellis et al. said that control measures implemented for the second outbreak included strict isolation, culling, increased sanitation and vaccination [34]. Antigenic analysis of the new avian isolates showed a reactivity pattern different from that of H5N1 viruses isolated in 1997 and 2001 [36]. This finding suggests that significant antigenic variation has recently occurred among H5N1 viruses [36].

Shortridge et al. noted that the poultry markets were of critical importance in the perpetuation and transmission of influenza viruses to other avian species and to mammals, including humans [32]. The transmission of avian H5N1 influenza viruses to 18 humans in Hong Kong in 1997 with six deaths established that avian influenza viruses can transmit to and cause lethal infection in humans [32, 37]. In February 2003, an avian H5N1 virus closely related to one of these viruses was isolated from two humans with acute respiratory distress, one of whom died [35]. Although A/Hong Kong/156/97 (H5N1/97)-like viruses associated with the "bird flu" incident in Hong Kong SAR have not been detected since the slaughter of poultry in 1997, its putative precursors continue to persist in the region [38]. Claas et al. said that H5N1 viruses isolated from humans by the end of 1997 lacked the ability to spread efficiently among humans and therefore had limited pandemic potential [39]. However, Zhou et al. demonstrated that the H5N1 viruses circulating in poultry comprised two distinguishable phylogenetic lineages in all genes that were in very rapid evolution [40]. According to Zhou et al., influenza viruses usually undergo rapid alteration of their surface glycoproteins, especially in the hemagglutinin, when introduced into new hosts [40]. Guan et al. said that the early detection of H5N1 viruses in the retail, live poultry markets led to preemptive intervention before the occurrence of human disease, but these newly emerging, highly pathogenic H5N1 viruses provide cause for pandemic concern [38].

Lau et al. said that in the event of a human-to-human H5N1 outbreak, the public in Hong Kong was likely to adopt preventive measures that may help contain the spread of the virus in the community [41]. For preventive measures, universal vaccination at local chicken farms was introduced in June 2003 and by the end of 2003 all chickens entering the live poultry markets in Hong Kong were vaccinated by killed H5N2 vaccine [42]. Ellis et al. reported in their observation on vaccination in Hong Kong that infection spread to the recently vaccinated sheds with low rates of H5N1 mortality in sheds when the chickens were between 9 and 18 days post-vaccination; however, after 18 days post-vaccination no more deaths from H5N1 avian influenza occurred and no evidence of asymptomatic shedding of the virus was detected [43]. In addition to vaccination, an enhanced biosecurity program on farms and in live poultry markets and a comprehensive surveillance program for poultry, wild birds, recreation park birds and pet birds were in place [42].

Bird Flu in Korea

Outbreaks of highly pathogenic avian influenza H5N1 in the Republic of Korea occurred in 2003/04 [44]. Farmed commercial ducks were the main affected animals. During the outbreak, the ducks developed clinical signs, including mild respiratory distress, depression, mild diarrhea, loss of appetite and increasing mortality [45]. Lee et al. reported that despite genetic similarities among recent H5N1 isolates, the topology of the phylogenetic tree clearly differentiated the Korean isolates from the Vietnamese and Thai isolates which had been reported to infect humans [46]. Lee et al. reported that a representative Korean isolate was inoculated into mice, with no mortality and no virus being isolated from the brain, although high titers of virus were observed in the lungs [46]. Mase et al. reported that the H5N1 viruses isolated in Korea and Japan were genetically similar at more than 99% identity in the nucleotide sequences of all eight RNA segments, indicating that they belonged to genotype V and were distinct from HPAI viruses prevalent in Southeast Asia that belonged to genotype Z [47]. According to another study by Yoon et al., the infection time and within-farm spread pattern of virus were analyzed for the highly pathogenic avian influenza outbreak on chicken farms using regression models based on epidemiological data [48]. Yoon et al. found that farmers recognized the abnormally high mortality resulting from HPAI approximately five days after infection [48]. Yoon et al. also reported that entire flocks would die within 12 days of introduction of the HPAI virus to the infected farm without any intervention [48].

Another outbreak of highly pathogenic avian influenza subtype H5N1 in broiler breeders occurred in Korea in 2005 [49]. Grossly, the dead breeders had lesions consistent with HPAI, including pancreatic mottling, splenomegaly, pulmonary edema and congestion, and hemorrhages in the mucosa of the proventriculus, gizzard and small intestine, and on the serosal surface [49]. This was the first report of an outbreak of HPAI in the chickens in South Korea [49]. In 2005, Kwon et al. reported a highly pathogenic avian influenza infection in magpies (*Pica pica sericea*) in South Korea [50]. Kwon et al. noted that the isolated virus was identified as a highly pathogenic H5N1, with hemagglutinin proteolytic cleavage site deduced amino acid sequence of QREKRKKR/GLFGAIAG [50]. This is the first report of HPAI in magpies [50].

In addition to highly pathogenic avian influenza H5N1, low pathogenic avian influenza is also reported in Korea. The first outbreak of low pathogenic avian influenza, H9N2 virus subtype, in 1996 prompted an eradication response, but low pathogenic avian influenza returned to Korea in 1999 [51]. Kwon et al. noted that phylogenetic analysis with internal genes showed that some Korean isolates formed a cluster with other subtypes, such as H5N1, H6N1, and H6N2 in China and Taiwan [51].

Bird Flu in Japan

There have been several emerging animal diseases and food-borne infection problems occurring in Japan over the last few years [52]. Yamane said that early detection of the first cases and rapid action in preventing and controlling the spread of infections were very important, combined with proper risk communication regarding the diseases [52]. In 2004, four cases of the highly pathogenic avian influenza (HPAI), which was the first outbreak after 79 years, and caused by the H5N1 subtype, were identified [52]. Highly pathogenic H5N1 avian influenza viruses were isolated in 9 large-billed crows that died in Kyoto and Osaka prefectures in Japan from March to April in 2004 [53]. The most prominent lesions were gross patchy areas of reddish discoloration in the pancreas and the consistent histologic lesions included severe multifocal necrotizing pancreatitis, focal degeneration and necrosis of neuron and glial cells in the central nervous system, and focal degeneration of cardiac myocytes [53]. In addition, an outbreak in hens was also reported [54]. Nakatani et al. reported that the farm, which had a total of 34,640 chickens, experienced up to 43.3% mortality before the chickens were depopulated [54]. According to report of Nakatani et al., the affected chickens exhibited mortality without apparent clinical signs [54]. Histologically, hepatocytic necrosis; necrosis of ellipsoids and follicles with fibrin in the spleen; necrosis with glial nodules in the brain stem, cerebrum, and cerebellum; necrosis of acinar cells in the pancreas; and necrosis of lymphoid tissues in intestinal lamina propria were seen [54]. During the outbreak of highly pathogenic avian influenza that occurred in Tamba Town, Kyoto Prefecture in 2004, a total of 926 flies were collected from six sites within a radius of 2.3 km from the poultry farm by Sawabe et al. [55]. Sawabe et al. suggested that it was possible that blow flies could become a mechanical transmitter of H5N1 influenza virus [55]. An H5N1 influenza A virus was isolated from duck meat processed for human consumption and imported to Japan from Shandong Province, China in 2003 [56]. Mase et al. said that poultry products contaminated with influenza viruses of high pathogenic potential to mammals were a threat to public health even in countries where the virus was not enzootic and represented a possible source of influenza outbreaks in poultry [56]. Mase et al. concluded that the H5N1 viruses associated with the influenza outbreaks in chickens in Japan were genotypically closely related to an H5N1 virus isolated from chicken in China in 2003 (genotype V), but were different from those prevalent in southeastern Asia in 2003-2004 (i.e., genotype Z) and that these highly pathogenic viruses could be transmitted to crows, which were highly susceptible to these viruses [57]. Anti-flu measures are a present focus in Japan [58]. Japan produced the "Pandemic Influenza Preparedness Action Plan" in 2005, and also took genuine measures against a new pathogenic avian influenza virus [59]. Yasui and Okabe said that the prevention of infection expansion, specification of the source of infection, assessment of the risk of infection, and early detection of new variant influenza virus and containment were expected by doing epidemiological investigations [60].

Bird Flu in Mongolia

Bird flu in Mongolia is not well described in the literature. However, the problem of H5N1 exists in this area. Chen et al. said that H5N1 viruses isolated in Mongolia, Russia, Inner Mongolia, and the Liaoning Province of China after August 2005 were genetically closely related to one of the genotypes isolated during the Qinghai outbreak, suggesting the dominant nature of this genotype and underscoring the need for worldwide intensive surveillance to minimize its devastating consequences [61]. Four influenza A viruses of the subtype H1N1, isolated from Mongolian patients in Ulaanbaatar between 1985 and 1991, were analyzed by the sequencing of various RNA segments [62]. Anchlan et al. reported that the isolate from 1985 was found to be highly related in all genes sequenced to strains isolated from camels in the same region and at about the same time [62]. Anchlan et al. mentioned that the mutational and evolutionary rates of the Mongolian strains seem to be significantly lower when compared to the rates of human influenza A strains isolated in other parts of the world [62]. For human infection in Mongolia, H5N1 infections were reported in 1982, 1983, 1986 and 1987 from children with acute respiratory diseases [63].

Bird Flu in Taiwan

In 2003, an avian influenza (AI) virus of H5N1 subtype (A/Duck/China/E319-2/03; Dk/CHN/E319-2/03) was isolated from a smuggled duck in Kinmen Island of Taiwan [64]. Lee et al. suggested that ducks infected with H5N1 avian influenza of a highly pathogenic pathotype showing no disease signs can carry the virus silently and that bird smuggling represents a serious risk for H5N1 highly pathogenic avian influenza transmission [64]. Tzeng and Yin studied Taiwan nurses' fears and professional obligations concerning possible human-to-human avian flu [65]. According to this work, nearly 42% of the nurses did not think that, if there were an outbreak of avian flu, their working hospitals would have sufficient infection control measures and equipment to prevent nosocomial infection in their working environment [65]. In addition, about 57% of the nurse participants indicated that they were willing to care for patients infected with avian influenza [65].

Bird Flu in China

China is a big area with problems caused by many new emerging infectious diseases, as previously mentioned. Since their reemergence in 2003, highly pathogenic avian influenza A (H5N1) viruses have been transmitted from poultry to humans, either by direct or indirect contact with infected birds, in several provinces of Mainland China, which has resulted in many cases of human infection and has created repercussions for the Chinese economy [66]. In 2004, 3 and 4 strains of avian influenza virus subtype H5N1 were isolated from waterfowl and chickens, respectively, in central People's Republic of China [67]. Oyana et al. used geographic information systems (GIS) techniques combined with statistical techniques to analyze the spatiotemporal variation of reported cases of avian influenza [68]. Although we observed a major northeast-southwest distribution of the avian influenza H5N1 cases, there was no significant spatiotemporal association in average "direction of advance" of these cases [68]. The finding from this study is very consistent with the major migratory bird routes in East Asia, but owing to weak surveillance and reporting systems in the region, the study findings warrant further evaluation [68]. Of interest, new important strains of H5N1 were continuously reported. In 2006, Normile reported a new H5N1 strain emerging in southern China [69]. In addition, He et al. reported amantadine resistance among H5N1 avian influenza viruses isolated in Northern China [70]. He et al. said that amantadine was used extensively in poultry farms in this area, which may be for one of reasons of the high amantadine-resistance incidence [70]. In addition to H5N1, other types of bird flu have recently emerged in China [71 – 73].

References

[1]   Bedard BG, Hunt T. The emerging animal health delivery system in the People's Republic of China. *Rev. Sci. Tech.* 2004 Apr;23(1):297-304.

[2]   Tanno S. Importance of National Institute of Infectious Diseases and Institutes of Public Health on control of infectious diseases in the new century. *Jpn. J. Infect. Dis.* 2002 Dec;55(6):181-2.

[3]   Okabe N. Amendment to the infectious disease control law. *Uirusu.* 2004 Dec;54(2):249-54.

[4]   Wong GW. Out of the East--emerging infections. *Paediatr. Respir. Rev.* 2006;7 Suppl 1:S229-31.

[5]   Pokrovskaia AV. Severe acute respiratory syndrome. *Ter Arkh.* 2007;79(3):66-70.

[6]   Okabe N. Severe acute respiratory syndrome (SARS). *Nippon Rinsho.* 2007 Mar 28;65 Suppl .3:44-7.

[7]   Muller MP, McGeer A. Severe acute respiratory syndrome (SARS) coronavirus. Semin *Respir. Crit. Care Med.* 2007 Apr;28(2):201-12.

[8]   Poon LL, Guan Y, Nicholls JM, Yuen KY, Peiris JS. The aetiology, origins, and diagnosis of severe acute respiratory syndrome. *Lancet Infect. Dis.* 2004 Nov;4(11):663-71.

[9]   Yam LY, Chen RC, Zhong NS. SARS: ventilatory and intensive care. *Respirology.* 2003 Nov;8 Suppl:S31-5.

[10] Poon LL. SARS and other coronaviruses in humans and animals. *Adv. Exp. Med .Biol.* 2006;581:457-62.

[11] Fontanet A. Lessons from SARS. *Presse Med.* 2007 Feb;36(2 Pt 2):299-302.

[12] Xie HZ, Nie J, Pan SS, Bai Y. An epidemiological investigation on injection related risk factors. *Zhonghua Liu Xing Bing Xue Za Zhi.* 2003 Mar;24(3):172-5.

[13] Epidemics. War on an old scourge. Tuberculosis is back and some nations are unable to restrain it. *Asiaweek.* 1995 Sep 29;:45-6.

[14] Law C. Early growth and chronic disease: a public health overview. *Matern. Child Nutr.* 2005 Jul;1(3):169-76.

[15] *United States. Department of State. Bureau of Public Affairs. ASEAN.* Backgr. Notes Ser. 1986 Apr;:1-8.

[16] Tian X. Sustainable development of population and resources. *Chin. J. Popul. Sci.* 1996;8(3):239-47.

[17] Diczfalusy E. The third age, the Third World and the third millennium. *Contraception.* 1996 Jan;53(1):1-7.

[18] Mandavilli A. China: open season. *Nature.* 2006 Jan 26;439(7075):382-3.

[19] Sheff B. Avian influenza: poised to launch a pandemic? *Nursing.* 2006 Jan;36(1):51-3.

[20] Woo PC, Lau SK, Yuen KY. Infectious diseases emerging from Chinese wet-markets: zoonotic origins of severe respiratory viral infections. *Curr. Opin. Infect. Dis.* 2006 Oct;19(5):401-7.

[21] Cockburn WC, Delon PJ, Ferreira W. Origin and progress of the 1968-69 Hong Kong influenza epidemic. *Bull. World Health Organ.* 1969;41(3):345-8.

[22] Buescher EL, Smith TJ, Zachary IH. Experience with Hong Kong influenza in tropical areas. *Bull. World Health Organ.* 1969;41(3):387-91.

[23] Chang WK. National influenza experience in Hong Kong, 1968. *Bull. World Health Organ.* 1969;41(3):349-51.

[24] White PC Jr. A2-Hong Kong-68. *Va. Med. Mon.* (1918). 1968 Oct;95(10):595-6.

[25] Hrabar A, Ugrcic I. A-2 Hong Kong influenza epidemic in Croatia in 1969-70. *Lijec. Vjesn.* 1972 Mar;94(3):125-31.

[26] Kundin WD. Hong Kong influenza. Serological, immunochemical and epidemiologic studies. *Taiwan Yi Xue Hui Za Zhi.* 1969 Nov 28;68(11):568-9.

[27] Davis LE, Caldwell GG, Lynch RE, Bailey RE, Chin TD. Hong Kong influenza: the epidemiologic features of a high school family study analyzed and compared with a similar study during the 1957 Asian influenza epidemic. *Am. J. Epidemiol.* 1970 Oct;92(4):240-7.

[28] Influenza: the Hong Kong virus. *WHO Chron.* 1968 Dec;22(12):528-9.

[29] Vastag B. Hong Kong flu still poses pandemic threat. *JAMA.* 2002 Nov 20;288(19):2391-5.

[30] Hong Kong influenza: the coming winter. *Med. J. Aust.* 1970 Feb 21;1(8):393-4.

[31] Kung NY, Morris RS, Perkins NR, Sims LD, Ellis TM, Bissett L, Chow M, Shortridge KF, Guan Y, Peiris MJ. Risk for infection with highly pathogenic influenza A virus (H5N1) in chickens, Hong Kong, 2002. *Emerg. Infect. Dis.* 2007 Mar;13(3):412-8.

[32] Shortridge KF, Zhou NN, Guan Y, Gao P, Ito T, Kawaoka Y, Kodihalli S, Krauss S, Markwell D, Murti KG, Norwood M, Senne D, Sims L, Takada A, Webster RG. Characterization of avian H5N1 influenza viruses from poultry in Hong Kong. *Virology.* 1998 Dec 20;252(2):331-42.

[33] Cauthen AN, Swayne DE, Schultz-Cherry S, Perdue ML, Suarez DL. Continued circulation in China of highly pathogenic avian influenza viruses encoding the hemagglutinin gene associated with the 1997 H5N1 outbreak in poultry and humans. *J. Virol.* 2000 Jul;74(14):6592-9.

[34] Ellis TM, Bousfield RB, Bissett LA, Dyrting KC, Luk GS, Tsim ST, Sturm-Ramirez K, Webster RG, Guan Y, Malik Peiris JS. Investigation of outbreaks of highly pathogenic H5N1 avian influenza in waterfowl and wild birds in Hong Kong in late 2002. *Avian Pathol.* 2004 Oct;33(5):492-505.

[35] Sturm-Ramirez KM, Ellis T, Bousfield B, Bissett L, Dyrting K, Rehg JE, Poon L, Guan Y, Peiris M, Webster RG. Reemerging H5N1 influenza viruses in Hong Kong in 2002 are highly pathogenic to ducks. *J. Virol.* 2004 May;78(9):4892-901.

[36] Sturm-Ramirez KM, Ellis T, Bousfield B, Bissett L, Dyrting K, Rehg JE, Poon L, Guan Y, Peiris M, Webster RG. Reemerging H5N1 influenza viruses in Hong Kong in 2002 are highly pathogenic to ducks. *J. Virol.* 2004 May;78(9):4892-901.

[37] Sims LD, Ellis TM, Liu KK, Dyrting K, Wong H, Peiris M, Guan Y, Shortridge KF. Avian influenza in Hong Kong 1997-2002. *Avian Dis.* 2003;47(3 Suppl):832-8.

[38] Guan Y, Peiris JS, Lipatov AS, Ellis TM, Dyrting KC, Krauss S, Zhang LJ, Webster RG, Shortridge KF. Emergence of multiple genotypes of H5N1 avian influenza viruses in Hong Kong SAR. *Proc. Natl. Acad. Sci. U S A.* 2002 Jun 25;99(13):8950-5.

[39] Claas EC, de Jong JC, van Beek R, Rimmelzwaan GF, Osterhaus AD. Human influenza virus A/HongKong/156/97 (H5N1) infection. *Vaccine.* 1998 May-Jun;16(9-10):977-8.

[40] Zhou NN, Shortridge KF, Claas EC, Krauss SL, Webster RG. Rapid evolution of H5N1 influenza viruses in chickens in Hong Kong. *J. Virol.* 1999 Apr;73(4):3366-74.

[41] Lau JT, Kim JH, Tsui HY, Griffiths S. Anticipated and current preventive behaviors in response to an anticipated human-to-human H5N1 epidemic in the Hong Kong Chinese general population. *BMC Infect. Dis.* 2007 Mar 15;7:18.

[42] Ellis TM, Sims LD, Wong HK, Wong CW, Dyrting KC, Chow KW, Leung C, Peiris JS. Use of avian influenza vaccination in Hong Kong. *Dev. Biol.* (Basel). 2006;124:133-43.

[43] Ellis TM, Leung CY, Chow MK, Bissett LA, Wong W, Guan Y, Malik Peiris JS. Vaccination of chickens against H5N1 avian influenza in the face of an outbreak interrupts virus transmission. *Avian Pathol.* 2004 Aug;33(4):405-12.

[44] Wee SH, Park CK, Nam HM, Kim CH, Yoon H, Kim SJ, Lee ES, Lee BY, Kim JH, Lee JH, Kim CS. Outbreaks of highly pathogenic avian influenza (H5N1) in the Republic of Korea in 2003/04. *Vet. Rec.* 2006 Mar 11;158(10):341-4.

[45] Kwon YK, Joh SJ, Kim MC, Sung HW, Lee YJ, Choi JG, Lee EK, Kim JH. Highly pathogenic avian influenza (H5N1) in the commercial domestic ducks of South Korea. *Avian Pathol.* 2005 Aug;34(4):367-70.

[46] Lee CW, Suarez DL, Tumpey TM, Sung HW, Kwon YK, Lee YJ, Choi JG, Joh SJ, Kim MC, Lee EK, Park JM, Lu X, Katz JM, Spackman E, Swayne DE, Kim JH. Characterization of highly pathogenic H5N1 avian influenza A viruses isolated from South Korea. *J. Virol.* 2005 Mar;79(6):3692-702.

[47] Mase M, Kim JH, Lee YJ, Tsukamoto K, Imada T, Imai K, Yamaguchi S. Genetic comparison of H5N1 influenza A viruses isolated from chickens in Japan and Korea. *Microbiol. Immunol.* 2005;49(9):871-4.

[48] Yoon H, Park CK, Nam HM, Wee SH. Virus spread pattern within infected chicken farms using regression model: the 2003-2004 HPAI epidemic in the Republic of Korea. *J. Vet. Med. B. Infect. Dis. Vet. Public Health.* 2005 Dec;52(10):428-31.

[49] Kwon YK, Joh SJ, Kim MC, Sung HW, Lee YJ, Choi JG, Lee EK, Kim JH. Highly pathogenic avian influenza (H5N1) in the commercial domestic ducks of South Korea. *Avian Pathol.* 2005 Aug;34(4):367-70.

[50] Kwon YK, Joh SJ, Kim MC, Lee YJ, Choi JG, Lee EK, Wee SH, Sung HW, Kwon JH, Kang MI, Kim JH. Highly pathogenic avian influenza in magpies (Pica pica sericea) in South Korea. *J. Wildl. Dis.* 2005 Jul;41(3):618-23.

[51] Kwon HJ, Cho SH, Kim MC, Ahn YJ, Kim SJ. Molecular epizootiology of recurrent low pathogenic avian influenza by H9N2 subtype virus in Korea. *Avian Pathol.* 2006 Aug;35(4):309-15.

[52] Yamane I. Epidemics of emerging animal diseases and food-borne infection problems over the last 5 years in Japan. *Ann. N Y Acad Sci.* 2006 Oct;1081:30-8.

[53] Tanimura N, Tsukamoto K, Okamatsu M, Mase M, Imada T, Nakamura K, Kubo M, Yamaguchi S, Irishio W, Hayashi M, Nakai T, Yamauchi A, Nishimura M, Imai K. Pathology of fatal highly pathogenic H5N1 avian influenza virus infection in large-billed crows (Corvus macrorhynchos) during the 2004 outbreak in Japan. *Vet. Pathol.* 2006 Jul;43(4):500-9.

[54] Nakatani H, Nakamura K, Yamamoto Y, Yamada M, Yamamoto Y. Epidemiology, pathology, and immunohistochemistry of layer hens naturally affected with H5N1 highly pathogenic avian influenza in Japan. *Avian Dis.* 2005 Sep;49(3):436-41.

[55] Sawabe K, Hoshino K, Isawa H, Sasaki T, Hayashi T, Tsuda Y, Kurahashi H, Tanabayashi K, Hotta A, Saito T, Yamada A, Kobayashi M. Detection and isolation of highly pathogenic H5N1 avian influenza A viruses from blow flies collected in the vicinity of an infected poultry farm in Kyoto, Japan, 2004. *Am. J. Trop. Med. Hyg.* 2006 Aug;75(2):327-32.

[56] Mase M, Eto M, Tanimura N, Imai K, Tsukamoto K, Horimoto T, Kawaoka Y, Yamaguchi S. Isolation of a genotypically unique H5N1 influenza virus from duck meat imported into Japan from China. *Virology.* 2005 Aug 15;339(1):101-9.

[57] Mase M, Tsukamoto K, Imada T, Imai K, Tanimura N, Nakamura K, Yamamoto Y, Hitomi T, Kira T, Nakai T, Kiso M, Horimoto T, Kawaoka Y, Yamaguchi S. Characterization of H5N1 influenza A viruses isolated during the 2003-2004 influenza outbreaks in Japan. *Virology.* 2005 Feb 5;332(1):167-76.

[58] Suzuki K, Hirota Y. Anti-flu measures in Japan. *Rev. Pneumol. Clin.* 2006 Sep;62(4):213-4.

[59] Nishijima Y, Umeda M. Pandemic influenza measures in Japan--from the point of government. *Nippon Rinsho.* 2006 Oct;64(10):1781-8.

[60] Yasui Y, Okabe N. Seasonal influenza activity in Japan and epidemiological investigation for avian influenza. *Uirusu.* 2006 Jun;56(1):67-75.

[61] Chen H, Li Y, Li Z, Shi J, Shinya K, Deng G, Qi Q, Tian G, Fan S, Zhao H, Sun Y, Kawaoka Y. Properties and dissemination of H5N1 viruses isolated during an influenza outbreak in migratory waterfowl in western China. *J. Virol.* 2006 Jun;80(12):5976-83.

[62] Anchlan D, Ludwig S, Nymadawa P, Mendsaikhan J, Scholtissek C. Previous H1N1 influenza A viruses circulating in the Mongolian population. *Arch. Virol.* 1996;141(8):1553-69.

[63] Iamnikova SS, Nimadava P, Petrov NA, Vasilenko SK, Iakhno MA, Semenova NP, L'vov DK. The characteristics of influenza A/H1N1 viruses related to A/PR/8/34 isolated in the Mongolian People's Republic. *Vopr. Virusol.* 1991 May-Jun;36(3):188-91.

[64] Lee MS, Deng MC, Lin YJ, Chang CY, Shieh HK, Shiau JZ, Huang CC. Characterization of an H5N1 avian influenza virus from Taiwan. *Vet. Microbiol.* 2007 Oct 6;124(3-4):193-201.

[65] Tzeng HM, Yin CY. Nurses' fears and professional obligations concerning possible human-to-human avian flu. Nurs Ethics. 2006 Sep;13(5):455-70.

[66] Su Z, Xu H, Chen J. Avian influenza: should China be alarmed? *Yonsei Med. J.* 2007 Aug 31;48(4):586-94.

[67] Yu Z. Avian Influenza (H5N1) Virus in Waterfowl and Chickens, Central China. *Emerg. Infect. Dis.* 2007 May;13(5):772-5.

[68] Oyana TJ, Dai D, Scott KE. Spatiotemporal distributions of reported cases of the avian influenza H5N1 (bird flu) in Southern China in early 2004. *Avian Dis.* 2006 Dec;50(4):508-15.

[69] Normile D. Avian influenza. New H5N1 strain emerges in southern China. *Science.* 2006 Nov 3;314(5800):742.

[70] He G, Qiao J, Dong C, He C, Zhao L, Tian Y. Amantadine-resistance among H5N1 avian influenza viruses isolated in Northern China. *Antiviral Res.* 2007 Sep 12;

[71]   Xu KM, Smith GJ, Bahl J, Duan L, Tai H, Vijaykrishna D, Wang J, Zhang JX, Li KS, Fan XH, Webster RG, Chen H, Peiris JS, Guan Y. Establishment of influenza A virus (H6N1) in minor poultry species in southern China. *J. Virol.* 2007 Oct;81(19):10402-12.

[72]   Cheung CL, Vijaykrishna D, Smith GJ, Fan XH, Zhang JX, Bahl J, Duan L, Huang K, Tai H, Wang J, Poon LL, Peiris JS, Chen H, Guan Y. Establishment of influenza A virus (H6N1) in minor poultry species in southern China. *J. Virol.* 2007 Oct;81(19):10402-12.

[73]   Serena Beato M, Terregino C, Cattoli G, Capua I. Isolation and characterization of an H10N7 avian influenza virus from poultry carcasses smuggled from China into Italy. *Avian Pathol.* 2006 Oct;35(5):400-3.

Chapter 3

Bird Flu in Southeast Asia

Bird Flu in Thailand [1 – 5]

In Thailand, the first confirmed H5N1 infection in avians was firstly reported on January 23, 2004. According to this sporadic episode, a control method of destroying all avians in the setting and in the surrounding 5-kilometers was established. In addition, a shoot count of avian transporting was done. The situation improved; however, a new episode occurred in July 2004. The second episode became pandemic. The Thai Prime Minister, Thaksin Shinawat, proposed an "X-ray scanning project" as a strict surveillance in all provinces of Thailand. This project started in October 2004 and was completed in November of the same year. In a recent study by Kaewcharoen et al., the hemagglutinin and neuraminidase genes of eight influenza A virus H5N1 isolates obtained from various avian species in Thailand in 2003-2004 was characterized in comparison with the Thai isolate A/Chicken/Nakorn-Pathom/Thailand/CU-K2/04(H5N1) [6]. According to this study, the amino acid sequence of the HA cleavage site revealed a common characteristic of a highly pathogenic virus strain [6]. Viseshakul et al. demonstrated that the Thai avian influenza emerged as a member of 2000's AI lineage with most of the genetic sequences closely related to the influenza A/Duck/China/E319.2/03 H5N1 [7]. A remission was derived. However, a third episode occurred again in July 2005. It should be noted that the second and third episodes might be the continuums of the first episode. Amonsin et al. reported that sequence analysis of eight gene segments revealed that the 2005 H5N1 viruses isolated in October 2005 were closely related to those recovered from chicken, tigers and humans in January and July 2004 [8]. The three peaks of occurrence might be due to the unawareness and under-detection of sick chicken by the avian farm managers and there might be a new significant epidemic outbreak of disease in chickens.

Buranathai et al. said that phylogenetic analysis revealed that Thai isolates were in the same cluster as Vietnamese isolates but aligned in a different cluster from Indonesian, Hong Kong, and Chinese viruses [9]. In addition, genetic analysis showed that most avian influenza virus isolates from Thailand had no major genetic changes in each gene such as HA (HA cleavage site, receptor binding site, N-link glycosylation site), NA (NA stalk region, oseltamivir resistance marker), M (the amantadine resistance marker, host specificity site),

NS (five amino acid deletion site), and PB2 (host specificity site) [9]. Buranathai et al. also reported that all Thai poultry isolates contained the amantadine resistance marker while none of them had the oseltamivir resistance marker [9].

In Thailand, human H5N1infection was first reported in the first outbreak in 2004 and could be detected in all other episodes [10 - 11]. Of the three episodes, there were 22 fatal human cases in total. In Thai infected cases, fever preceded dyspnea by a median of five days, and lymphopenia significantly predicted acute respiratory distress syndrome development and death [11]. Chotpitayasunondh et al. said that a history of direct contact with sick poultry, young age, pneumonia and lymphopenia, and progression to acute respiratory distress syndrome should prompt specific laboratory testing for H5N1 influenza [11]. Puthavathana et al. reported that all genomic segments of the Thailand human H5N1 influenza viruses clustered with the recently described genotype Z [12]. Puthavathana et al. also reported that the Thailand human H5N1 influenza viruses contained more avian-specific residues than the 1997 Hong Kong H5N1 viruses, suggesting that the virus might have adapted to allow a more efficient spread in avian species [12]. Probable person-to-person transmission of avian influenza A H5N1 was also first reported in Thailand by Ungchusak et al. [13]. The index patient became ill three to four days after her last exposure to dying household chickens. Her mother came from a distant city to care for her in the hospital, had no recognized exposure to poultry, and died from pneumonia after providing 16 to 18 hours of unprotected nursing care [13]. Of interest, Apisarnthanarak et al. studied the seroprevalence of anti-H5 antibody among Thai health care workers after exposure to avian influenza H5N1 in a tertiary care center [14]. Apisanthanarak et al. found that there was no serological evidence reactivity or subclinical infection in the studied population [14]. The possibility of human to human transmission of H5N1 infection is still a controversial issue.

The human bird flu infection became a new emergency disease under control of the Thai Center of Disease Control (CDC). In addition, the Thai government set up a center to cope with the problem of bird flu. A protocol to destroy all avians in a five kilometer area of suspected avian death due to H5N1 infection and strict surveillance in fifty kilometer area was implemented.

Not only humans and avians but also other animals were infected with H5N1 in the third outbreak. There were interesting reports of tiger and leopard infections in a tiger farm in Sriracha district near Pattaya, a famous breach of Thailand. Kaewcharoen et al. demonstrated that avian influenza A (H5N1) virus caused severe pneumonia in tigers and leopards that fed on infected poultry carcasses [15]. The H5N1 avian influenza virus outbreak among zoo tigers in mid-October 2004, with 45 animals dead, indicated that the avian influenza virus could cause lethal infection in a large mammalian species other than humans [16]. Amonsin et al. noted that sequence analyses also showed that the tiger H5N1 isolated in October 2004 was more closely related to the chicken H5N1 isolated in July than that from January [16]. A probable horizontal transmission among tigers was also demonstrated in this tiger zoo [17]. Recently, Kuiken et al. experimentally inoculated cats with H5N1 virus intratracheally and by feeding them virus-infected chickens [18]. According to this work, the cats excreted virus, developed severe diffuse alveolar damage, and transmitted virus to sentinel cats [18]. Kuiken et al. concluded that these results showed that domestic cats were at risk of disease or death from H5N1 virus, could be infected by horizontal transmission, and may play a role in the epidemiology of this virus [18].

Due to the three-peak pattern episode of H5N1, infection in Thailand, bird flu has become a new dangerous disease for the Thai people. Surveillance is continuously done [19]. Many rumors of bird flu spread throughout in Thailand. Panic symptoms [20 - 27] are commonly presented to the physicians. A health education to general population was set. Olsen et al. surveyed residents of rural Thailand regarding avian influenza knowledge, attitudes, and practices and suggested that public education campaigns had been effective in reaching those at greatest risk, although some high-risk behavior continues [28]. A report on bird flu was prepared by Thai researchers. During the three peak episodes, millions of chicken in Thailand were killed and this affected the Thai economy. People were afraid to ingest chicken forcing chicken farmers to close their businesses. In addition, avian to human infection in Thailand became a global concern. An anticipated global epidemic is a big threat to human beings. Luckily, there is no human epidemic at present.

As previously mentioned, human H5N1 cases have been reported since the first H5N1 episode in Thailand in 2004. The first two human cases in Thailand were children living in Kanchanaburi and Suphanburi provinces in Central Regions of Thailand. These two children had a history of close contact to the sick domestic chickens owned by in their families. They played and lived with infected chicken cases. At first, these two children were diagnosed as simple flu, but their symptoms were abruptly progressive. Finally, these two children died. In the first episode in 2004, there was a total of 10 human H5N1 cases and eight died. In the second episode, there were an additional five human infected cases with four deaths. In the third and last episode in 2005, five human cases could be detected. However, the fatality decreased; only two people died. This implies a good management program and use of antiviral drugs.

Table 1. A summary of important events during the three peak episode of H5N1, infection in Thailand

Episode	Details
1	This episode occurred during January to May 2004 (23 Jan 04-24 May 04). There were 181 foci of avian H5N1, infection in 41 provinces of Thailand. One hundred and forty-one sub-districts in Thailand were affected in this episode. The Central region of Thailand was believed to be the first focus or source of distribution. Farm chickens were the main affected animals.
2	The episode occurred during July to November 2004. There were 206 foci in 35 provinces. A larger area of H5N1 spreading than the first episode could be identified. This episode covered 789 sub-districts of Thailand. All regions of Thailand were affected. The main affected animals were farm chickens. During this episode millions of chickens were killed. Many chicken farms were bankrupted. Chicken product from Thailand was banned. It is estimated that sixty billion bahts (about two billion US dollar) lost on to this crisis.

Table 1. (Continued).

3	This episode was identified in July 2005. This was not as large as the first and second episodes due to a well-prepared sector to cope with the problem in Thailand. The situation was relieved in early 2006. Similar to the first and the
	Thailand. The situation was relieved in early 2006. Similar to the first and the second outbreaks, human infection can be seen. The concern regarding human H5N1 infection created a widespread bird flu panic among Thai people.

Table 2. A summary of human H5N1 infection and mortality in Thailand.

Period	Number*	
	Infection	Death
Dec 03 – Mar 04	12	8
Jul 04 – Oct 04	5	4
Dec 04 – Oct 05	5	2

*All are confirmed infected cases according to the WHO definition (positive influenza A H5N1 culture and/or positive H5 by RT-PCR method and/a positive 4 –fold rising of H5-specific antibody).

Bird Flu in Vietnam [29 – 41]

Vietnam is another country in Southeast Asia which with the problem of recent H5N1 epidemics. The epidemic started in early 2004. In 2004, Tran et al. reported 10 cases of H5N1 infected Vietnamese [42]. In all 10 cases the infection appeared to have been acquired directly from infected poultry; the potential existed for genetic reassortment with human influenza viruses and the evolution of human-to-human transmission [42]. Dinh et al. performed a study to evaluate risk factors for human infection with influenza A subtype H5N1 by a matched case-control study technique [43]. Dinh et al. noted that factors not significantly associated with infection were raising healthy poultry, preparing healthy poultry for consumption, and exposure to persons with an acute respiratory illness [43]. In 2006, Muramoto et al. took viruses isolated from poultry and humans in Vietnam and tested their virulence in mice [44]. The results showed that the H5N1 viruses from humans were pathogenic in mice and that one avian isolate was also pathogenic [44]. Muramoto et al. said that the H5N1 viruses circulating in poultry adapted during replication in humans or that strains pathogenic in mice were transmitted directly to humans [44]. Muramoto et al. molecularly characterized the hemagglutinin and neuraminidase genes of nine H5N1 viruses isolated between January 2004 and August 2005 from domestic poultry in Vietnam [45]. Muramoto et al. found that several groups of highly pathogenic H5N1 avian influenza viruses have been circulating among these birds, which suggests that H5N1 viruses of different lineages have been introduced into Vietnam multiple times [45].

Nguyen et al. conducted an interesting cross-sectional virologic study in live bird markets (LBM) in Hanoi, Vietnam, in October 2001 [46]. According to this work, the results established that HP H5N1 viruses with properties similar to viruses isolated in Hong Kong and mainland China circulated in Vietnam as early as 2001, suggested a common source for H5N1 viruses circulating in these Asian countries, and provided a framework to better understand the recent widespread emergence of HP H5N1 viruses in Asia [46]. In 2006, Li et al. reported that three H5N1 influenza viruses were isolated from shell washes of duck and goose eggs confiscated from travelers coming from Vietnam [47]. Although the source of these recently isolated Hong Kong 97-like H5N1 viruses is undetermined, Li et al. said that their detection in the egg shells of ducks and geese suggested that this particular genotype of H5N1 virus might have re-emerged in nature or may have been circulating continuously [47].

Responding to the epidemic of bird flu in Vietnam, similar control processes to those of Thailand were implemented. After a consultancy mission was funded by a nongovernmental organization (NGO), Cristalli and Capua collected information on the dynamics of avian influenza infection at the rural level in a Vietnamese province with several ongoing outbreaks [48]. On the basis of the data collected during the mission, particularly on rural and semi-intensive poultry rearing systems, *Cristalli* and *Capua* proposed that the application of an effective vaccination strategy including backyard flocks coupled with dissemination of relevant information on biosecurity measures should be developed for decision makers [48].

Another important point of concern is the high rate of drug-resistant H5N1 virus reported in Vietnam [49]. In 2005, Le et al. first reported the isolation of an H5N1 virus from a Vietnamese girl that was resistant to the drug oseltamivir, which was an inhibitor of the viral enzyme neuraminidase used for protection against and treatment of influenza [50]. Finding a new anti-H5N1 drug is the main focus of present bird flu research [51].

Bird Flu in Cambodia [52 – 56]

Cambodia is also affected by the emergence of H5N1 [57]. Cambodia has had 15 confirmed highly pathogenic avian influenza (H5N1) outbreaks in different sectors of the poultry industry since January 2004 [58]. Buchy et al. reported clinical aspects of human H5N1 infection in Cambodia [59]. Buchy reported that the high frequency of virus isolation from serum and faecal swabs highlights that H5N1 was likely to be a disseminated infection in humans and that this had implications for antiviral treatment, biosafety in clinical laboratories and on risks for nosocomial and human-to-human transmission; however, there were no tissue-specific adaptive mutations in the hemagglutinin gene from viruses isolated from different organs [59]. Of interest, Vong et al. noted low frequency of poultry-to-human H5NI virus transmission in southern Cambodia in 2005 [60]. Vong et al. reported that despite frequent, direct contact with poultry suspected of having H5N1 virus infection, none of villagers in the epidemic areas had neutralizing antibodies to H5N1 [60].

Because Cambodia has very limited human and financial resources, when the outbreak first began, the veterinary services were not equipped with the basic tools to collect accurate epidemiological information or to fight the disease [58]. Therefore, different agencies, under the umbrella of the Food and Agriculture Organisation, are providing support to the Cambodian Government to strengthen its capacity to diagnose, survey and control the avian influenza virus [58]. Emergency assistance in laboratory development for control of avian influenza in Laos and Cambodia was launched from many Western countries [61].

Responding to the epidemic of bird flu in Cambodia, control processes similar to those of Thailand and Vietnam were established. In 2007, Ly et al. conducted a knowledge, attitudes, and practices survey of poultry-handling behavior among villagers in rural Cambodia [62]. According to this work, despite widespread knowledge of avian influenza and personal protection measures, most rural Cambodians still maintained a high level of at-risk poultry handling [62].

Bird Flu in Indonesia [63 - 79]

Recently, bird flu emerged in Indonesia and became the new focus of a H5N1 world. Highly pathogenic avian influenza A H5N1 virus was detected in domestic poultry in Indonesia beginning in 2003 and is now widespread among backyard poultry flocks in many provinces [80]. The first human case of H5N1 virus infection in Indonesia was identified in July 2005 [80]. Sporadic and family clusters of cases of H5N1 virus infection, with a high case-fatality proportion, occurred throughout Indonesia during 2005-2006 [80]. Smith et al. said that H5N1 viruses had evolved over time into geographically distinct groups within Indonesia and Vietnam [81]. Smith et al. noted that molecular analysis of the H5N1 genotype Z genome showed that only the M2 and PB1-F2 genes were under positive selection, suggesting that these genes might be involved in adaptation of this virus to new hosts following interspecies transmission [81]. They also provided a new finding on the ongoing evolution of H5N1 influenza viruses that are transmitting in diverse avian species and at the interface between avian and human hosts [81].

Bird Flu in Laos

Similar to Cambodia, H5N1 infection is also reported in Laos, another poor developing country in Southeast Asia. The disease was firstly detected in 2002. Boltz et al. reported isolation of H5N1 virus genetically distinct from H5N1 circulating in 2004, which indicated reintroduction of H5N1 into Lao PDR after its disappearance for 2 years [82]. For disease control, a prospective surveillance program for influenza viruses was established in Lao PDR in July of 2005 [82 - 83].

Bird Flu in Other Countries in Southeast Asia

Of interest, although bird flu infections have been reported in many countries in Southeast Asia, there are no reports from Malaysia, Brunei or Singparore. This might reflect good disease control processes in these three countries. There is no report from Myanmar as well. However, the reason might due to the blockage of data by the Myanmar government or poor ability to detect the disease within Myanmar.

References

[1]   Tiensin T, Chaitaweesub P, Songserm T, Chaisingh A, Hoonsuwan W, Buranathai C, Parakamawongsa T, Premashthira S, Amonsin A, Gilbert M, Nielen M, Stegeman A. Highly pathogenic avian influenza H5N1, Thailand, 2004. *Emerg. Infect. Dis.* 2005 Nov;11(11):1664-72.

[2]   Lipatov AC, Smirnov IuA, Kaverin NV, Webster RG. Evolution of avian influenza viruses H5N1 (1997-2004) in southern and south-eastern Asia. *Vopr. Virusol.* 2005 Jul-Aug;50(4):11-7.

[3]   Tiensin T, Nielen M, Songserm T, Kalpravidh W, Chaitaweesub P, Amonsin A, Chotiprasatintara S, Chaisingh A, Damrongwatanapokin S, Wongkasemjit S, Antarasena C, Songkitti V, Chanachai K, Thanapongtham W, Stegeman JA.Geographic and temporal distribution of highly pathogenic avian influenza A virus (H5N1) in Thailand, 2004-2005: an overview. *Avian Dis.* 2007 Mar;51(1 Suppl):182-8.

[4]   Songserm T, Jam-on R, Sae-Heng N, Meemak N, Hulse-Post DJ, Sturm-Ramirez KM, Webster RG. Domestic ducks and H5N1 influenza epidemic, Thailand. *Emerg. Infect Dis.* 2006 Apr;12(4):575-81.

[5]   Buranathai C, Amonsin A, Chaisigh A, Theamboonlers A, Pariyothorn N, Poovorawan Y. Surveillance activities and molecular analysis of H5N1 highly pathogenic avian influenza viruses from Thailand, 2004-2005. *Avian Dis.* 2007 Mar;51(1 Suppl):194-200.

[6]   Keawcharoen J, Amonsin A, Oraveerakul K, Wattanodorn S, Papravasit T, Karnda S, Lekakul K, Pattanarangsan R, Noppornpanth S, Fouchier RA, Osterhaus AD, Payungporn S, Theamboonlers A, Poovorawan Y. Characterization of the hemagglutinin and neuraminidase genes of recent influenza virus isolates from different avian species in Thailand. *Acta Virol.* 2005;49(4):277-80.

[7]   Viseshakul N, Thanawongnuwech R, Amonsin A, Suradhat S, Payungporn S, Keawchareon J, Oraveerakul K, Wongyanin P, Plitkul S, Theamboonlers A, Poovorawan Y. The genome sequence analysis of H5N1 avian influenza A virus isolated from the outbreak among poultry populations in Thailand. *Virology.* 2004 Oct 25;328(2):169-76.

[8]   Amonsin A, Chutinimitkul S, Pariyothorn N, Songserm T, Damrongwantanapokin S, Puranaveja S, Jam-On R, Sae-Heng N, Payungporn S, Theamboonlers A, Chaisingh A, Tantilertcharoen R, Suradhat S, Thanawongnuwech R, Poovorawan Y. Genetic characterization of influenza A viruses (H5N1) isolated from 3rd wave of Thailand AI outbreaks. *Virus Res.* 2006 Dec;122(1-2):194-9.

[9]   Buranathai C, Amonsin A, Chaisigh A, Theamboonlers A, Pariyothorn N, Poovorawan Y. Surveillance activities and molecular analysis of H5N1 highly pathogenic avian influenza viruses from Thailand, 2004-2005. *Avian Dis.* 2007 Mar;51(1 Suppl):194-200.

[10] Lye DC, Ang BS, Leo YS. Review of human infections with avian influenza H5N1 and proposed local clinical management guideline. *Ann. Acad. Med. Singapore.* 2007 Apr;36(4):285-92.

[11] Chotpitayasunondh T, Ungchusak K, Hanshaoworakul W, Chunsuthiwat S, Sawanpanyalert P, Kijphati R, Lochindarat S, Srisan P, Suwan P, Osotthanakorn Y, Anantasetagoon T, Kanjanawasri S, Tanupattarachai S, Weerakul J, Chaiwirattana R, Maneerattanaporn M, Poolsavathitikool R, Chokephaibulkit K, Apisarnthanarak A, Dowell SF. Human disease from influenza A (H5N1), Thailand, 2004. *Emerg. Infect. Dis.* 2005 Feb;11(2):201-9.

[12] Puthavathana P, Auewarakul P, Charoenying PC, Sangsiriwut K, Pooruk P, Boonnak K, Khanyok R, Thawachsupa P, Kijphati R, Sawanpanyalert P. Molecular characterization of the complete genome of human influenza H5N1 virus isolates from Thailand. *J. Gen. Virol.* 2005 Feb;86(Pt 2):423-33.

[13] Ungchusak K, Auewarakul P, Dowell SF, Kitphati R, Auwanit W, Puthavathana P, Uiprasertkul M, Boonnak K, Pittayawonganon C, Cox NJ, Zaki SR, Thawatsupha P, Chittaganpitch M, Khontong R, Simmerman JM, Chunsutthiwat S. Probable person-to-person transmission of avian influenza A (H5N1). *N. Engl. J. Med.* 2005 Jan 27;352(4):333-40.

[14] Apisarnthanarak A, Erb S, Stephenson I, Katz JM, Chittaganpitch M, Sangkitporn S, Kitphati R, Thawatsupha P, Waicharoen S, Pinitchai U, Apisarnthanarak P, Fraser VJ, Mundy LM. Seroprevalence of anti-H5 antibody among Thai health care workers after exposure to avian influenza (H5N1) in a tertiary care center. *Clin. Infect. Dis.* 2005 Jan 15;40(2):e16-8.

[15] Keawcharoen J, Oraveerakul K, Kuiken T, Fouchier RA, Amonsin A, Payungporn S, Noppornpanth S, Wattanodorn S, Theambooniers A, Tantilertcharoen R, Pattanarangsan R, Arya N, Ratanakorn P, Osterhaus DM, Poovorawan Y. Avian influenza H5N1 in tigers and leopards. *Emerg. Infect. Dis.* 2004 Dec;10(12):2189-91.

[16] Amonsin A, Payungporn S, Theamboonlers A, Thanawongnuwech R, Suradhat S, Pariyothorn N, Tantilertcharoen R, Damrongwantanapokin S, Buranathai C, Chaisingh A, Songserm T, Poovorawan Y. Genetic characterization of H5N1 influenza A viruses isolated from zoo tigers in Thailand. *Virology.* 2006 Jan 20;344(2):480-91.

[17] Thanawongnuwech R, Amonsin A, Tantilertcharoen R, Damrongwatanapokin S, Theamboonlers A, Payungporn S, Nanthapornphiphat K, Ratanamungklanon S, Tunak E, Songserm T, Vivatthanavanich V, Lekdumrongsak T, Kesdangsakonwut S, Tunhikorn S, Poovorawan Y. Probable tiger-to-tiger transmission of avian influenza H5N1. *Emerg. Infect. Dis.* 2005 May;11(5):699-701.

[18] Kuiken T, Rimmelzwaan G, van Riel D, van Amerongen G, Baars M, Fouchier R, Osterhaus A. Avian H5N1 influenza in cats. *Science.* 2004 Oct 8;306(5694):241.

[19] Olsen SJ, Ungchusak K, Birmingham M, Bresee J, Dowell SF, Chunsuttiwat S. Surveillance for avian influenza in human beings in Thailand. *Lancet Infect Dis.* 2006 Dec;6(12):757-8.

[20] Moscioni S. Stricken by panic or bird seed? Recenti Prog Med. 2005 Nov;96(11):559.

[21] Basu P. Panic over bird flu pandemic premature, experts say. *Nat. Med.* 2006 Mar;12(3):258.

[22] Bonneux L, Van Damme W. An iatrogenic pandemic of panic. *BMJ.* 2006 Apr 1;332(7544):786-8.

[23] Bird flu: don't fly into a panic. Whether the H5N1 virus will "make the jump" and spread among humans is uncertain, but here are some tips to protect yourself. *Harv. Health Lett.* 2006 Jun;31(8):1-3.

[24] Richards G. Avian influenza: preparation not panic. *Prim. Care Respir. J.* 2006 Aug;15(4):217-8.

[25] Nau JY. Washington's state of panic: 200 million dollars. *Rev. Med. Suisse.* 2006 Dec 6;2(90):2825.

[26] Kmietowicz Z. Political lead essential to avoid panic when flu strikes. *BMJ.* 2005 Nov 12;331(7525):1099.

[27] Manderscheid RW. reparing for pandemic Avian influenza: ensuring mental health services and mitigating panic. *Arch. Psychiatr. Nurs.* 2007 Feb;21(1):64-7.

[28] Olsen SJ, Laosiritaworn Y, Pattanasin S, Prapasiri P, Dowell SF. Poultry-handling practices during avian influenza outbreak, Thailand. *Emerg Infect Dis.* 2005 Oct;11(10):1601-3.

[29] Avian influenza, Viet Nam--update. *Wkly Epidemiol Rec.* 2005 Jul 8;80(27):233-4.

[30] Normile D. Avian influenza. Vietnam battles bird flu ... and critics. *Science.* 2005 Jul 15;309(5733):368-73.

[31] Avian influenza, Vietnam--update. *Can. Commun. Dis. Rep.* 2005 Jun 1;31(11):131.

[32] Avian influenza--Viet Nam and Cambodia--update. *Wkly. Epidemiol. Rec.* 2005 Apr 1;80(13):113-4.

[33] Avian influenza, Vietnam--update. *Can .Commun. Dis. Rep.* 2005 May 1;31(9):100-1.

[34] Avian influenza, Vietnam. *Can. Commun. Dis. Rep.* 2005 Mar 15;31(6):71.

[35] Avian influenza, Viet Nam--update. *Wkly Epidemiol. Rec.* 2005 Mar 18;80(11):93-4.

[36] Avian influenza, Vietnam. *Can. Commun. Dis. Rep.* 2005 Mar 1;31(5):64.

[37] Avian influenza, Viet Nam--update. *Wkly Epidemiol. Rec.* 2005 Feb 4;80(5):41-2.

[38] Infectious disease: Vietnam's war on flu. *Nature.* 2005 Jan 13;433(7022):102-4.

[39] Avian influenza--situation in Viet Nam as of 18 August 2004. *Wkly Epidemiol. Rec.* 2004 Aug 20;79(34):309.

[40] Avian influenza A(H5N1) in humans and poultry, Vietnam. *Wkly Epidemiol. Rec.* 2004 Jan 16;79(3):13-4.

[41] Parry J. WHO confirms avian flu outbreak in Hanoi. *BMJ.* 2004 Jan 17;328(7432):123.

[42] Tran TH, Nguyen TL, Nguyen TD, Luong TS, Pham PM, Nguyen VC, Pham TS, Vo CD, Le TQ, Ngo TT, Dao BK, Le PP, Nguyen TT, Hoang TL, Cao VT, Le TG, Nguyen DT, Le HN, Nguyen KT, Le HS, Le VT, Christiane D, Tran TT, Menno de J, Schultsz C, Cheng P, Lim W, Horby P, Farrar J; World Health Organization International Avian Influenza Investigative Team. Avian influenza A (H5N1) in 10 patients in Vietnam. *N. Engl. J. Med.* 2004 Mar 18;350(12):1179-88.

[43] Dinh PN, Long HT, Tien NT, Hien NT, Mai le TQ, Phong le H, Tuan le V, Van Tan H, Nguyen NB, Van Tu P, Phuong NT; World Health Organization/Global Outbreak Alert and Response Network Avian Influenza Investigation Team in Vietnam. Risk factors for human infection with avian influenza A H5N1, Vietnam, 2004. *Emerg. Infect. Dis.* 2006 Dec;12(12):1841-7.

[44] Muramoto Y, Le TQ, Phuong LS, Nguyen T, Nguyen TH, Sakai-Tagawa Y, Horimoto
      T, Kida H, Kawaoka Y. Pathogenicity of H5N1 influenza A viruses isolated in Vietnam
      between late 2003 and 2005. *J. Vet. Med. Sci.* 2006 Jul;68(7):735-7.

[45] Muramoto Y, Le TQ, Phuong LS, Nguyen T, Nguyen TH, Sakai-Tagawa Y, Iwatsuki-
      Horimoto K, Horimoto T, Kida H, Kawaoka Y. Molecular characterization of the
      hemagglutinin and neuraminidase genes of H5N1 influenza A viruses isolated from
      poultry in Vietnam from 2004 to 2005. *J. Vet. Med. Sci.* 2006 May;68(5):527-31.

[46] Nguyen DC, Uyeki TM, Jadhao S, Maines T, Shaw M, Matsuoka Y, Smith C, Rowe T,
      Lu X, Hall H, Xu X, Balish A, Klimov A, Tumpey TM, Swayne DE, Huynh LP,
      Nghiem HK, Nguyen HH, Hoang LT, Cox NJ, Katz JM. Isolation and characterization
      of avian influenza viruses, including highly pathogenic H5N1, from poultry in live bird
      markets in Hanoi, Vietnam, in 2001. *J. Virol.* 2005 Apr;79(7):4201-12.

[47] Li Y, Lin Z, Shi J, Qi Q, Deng G, Li Z, Wang X, Tian G, Chen H. Detection of Hong
      Kong 97-like H5N1 influenza viruses from eggs of Vietnamese waterfowl. *Arch. Virol.*
      2006 Aug;151(8):1615-24.

[48] Cristalli A, Capua I. Practical problems in controlling H5N1 high pathogenicity avian
      influenza at village level in Vietnam and introduction of biosecurity measures. *Avian
      Dis.* 2007 Mar;51(1 Suppl):461-2.

[49] ECDC Influenza Team. H5N1 virus resistant to oseltamivir isolated from Vietnamese
      patient. *Euro Surveill.* 2005 Oct 20;10(10):E051020.2.

[50] Le QM, Kiso M, Someya K, Sakai YT, Nguyen TH, Nguyen KH, Pham ND, Ngyen
      HH, Yamada S, Muramoto Y, Horimoto T, Takada A, Goto H, Suzuki T, Suzuki Y,
      Kawaoka Y. Avian flu: isolation of drug-resistant H5N1 virus. *Nature.* 2005 Oct
      20;437(7062):1108.

[51] Wiwanitkit V. Current research on drugs and vaccines for fighting bird flu. *Trans. R.
      Soc. Trop. Med. Hyg.* 2007 Jul 24;

[52] Morris SK. H5N1 avian influenza, Kampot Province, Cambodia. *Emerg. Infect. Dis.*
      2006 Jan;12(1):170-1.

[53] Outbreak news. Avian influenza, Cambodia. *Wkly Epidemiol. Rec.* 2006 Mar
      31;81(13):117.

[54] Officials report first Cambodian case of avian flu. *BMJ.* 2005 Feb 5;330(7486):273.

[55] Avian influenza, Cambodia--update. *Wkly Epidemiol. Rec.* 2005 Apr 15;80(15):133-4

[56] Influenza team, European Centre for Disease Prevention and Control. Evidence that
      mild or asymptomatic human H5N1 infections have no

[57] t occurred in a Cambodian village with poultry infections. *Euro Surveill.* 2006 Sep
      7;11(9):E060907.2.

[58] Suzuki JH. Human influenza--recent outbreak of avian influenza A/H5N1 among
      human in Asian countries--. *Nippon Rinsho.* 2005 Dec;63(12):2103-7.

[59] Desvaux S, Sorn S, Holl D, Chavernac D, Goutard F, Thonnat J, Porphyre V, Menard
      C, Cardinale E, Roger F. HPAI surveillance program in Cambodia: results and
      perspectives. *Dev. Biol* (Basel). 2006;124:211-24.

[60] Buchy P, Mardy S, Vong S, Toyoda T, Aubin JT, Miller M, Touch S, Sovann L,
      Dufourcq JB, Richner B, Tu PV, Tien NT, Lim W, Peiris JS, Van der Werf S. Influenza
      A/H5N1 virus infection in humans in Cambodia. *J. Clin. Virol.* 2007 Jul;39(3):164-8.

[61] Vong S, Coghlan B, Mardy S, Holl D, Seng H, Ly S, Miller MJ, Buchy P, Froehlich Y, Dufourcq JB, Uyeki TM, Lim W, Sok T. Low frequency of poultry-to-human H5NI virus transmission, southern Cambodia, 2005. *Emerg. Infect. Dis.* 2006 Oct;12(10):1542-7.

[62] Lu H. Emergency assistance in laboratory development for control of avian influenza in Laos and Cambodia. *Avian Dis.* 2007 Mar;51(1 Suppl):359-62.

[63] Ly S, Van Kerkhove MD, Holl D, Froehlich Y, Vong S. Interaction between humans and poultry, rural Cambodia. *Emerg. Infect. Dis.* 2007 Jan;13(1):130-2.

[64] Outbreak news. Avian influenza, Indonesia--update. *Wkly Epidemiol. Rec.* 2006 Oct 20;81(42):397.

[65] Avian influenza, Indonesia--update. *Wkly Epidemiol. Rec.* 2006 Oct 6;81(40):373.

[66] Outbreak news. Avian influenza, Indonesia--update. *Wkly Epidemiol. Rec.* 2006 Sep 15;81(37):349.

[67] Outbreak news. Avian influenza, Indonesia--update. *Wkly Epidemiol. Rec.* 2006 Jun 16;81(24):237.

[68] Outbreak news. Avian influenza, Indonesia--update. *Wkly Epidemiol. Rec.* 2006 Jun 9;81(23):233.

[69] Parry J. Failure to tackle flu in birds threatens Indonesia's human population. *BMJ.* 2006 Jun 10;332(7554):1354.

[70] Outbreak news. Avian influenza, Indonesia--update. *Wkly Epidemiol. Rec.* 2006 May 12;81(19):189.

[71] Outbreak news. Avian influenza, Indonesia--update. *Wkly Epidemiol. Rec.* 2006 Jan 27;81(4):33-4.

[72] Outbreak news. Avian influenza, Indonesia--update. *Wkly Epidemiol. Rec.* 2006 Feb 24;81(8):70-1.

[73] Outbreak news. Avian influenza, Indonesia--update. *Wkly Epidemiol. Rec.* 2006 Jan 6;81(1):2.

[74] Outbreak news. Avian influenza, Indonesia. *Wkly Epidemiol. Rec.* 2006 Jan 20;81(3):21.

[75] Outbreak news. Avian influenza, Indonesia--update. *Wkly Epidemiol. Rec.* 2006 Feb 10;81(6):49-50.

[76] Outbreak news. Avian influenza, Indonesia--update. *Wkly Epidemiol. Rec.* 2006 Feb 17;81(7):62.

[77] Butler D. Indonesia struggles to control bird flu outbreak. *Nature.* 2005 Oct 13;437(7061):937.

[78] World Health Organization. Avian influenza, Indonesia--update. *Wkly Epidemiol. Rec.* 2005 Oct 7;80(40):341-2.

[79] Avian influenza, Indonesia. *Wkly Epidemiol. Rec.* 2005 Sep 23;80(38):321-2.

[80] WHO confirms four human cases of avian flu in Indonesia. *BMJ.* 2005 Oct 8;331(7520):796.

[81] Sedyaningsih ER, Isfandari S, Setiawaty V, Rifati L, Harun S, Purba W, Imari S, Giriputra S, Blair PJ, Putnam SD, Uyeki TM, Soendoro T. Epidemiology of cases of H5N1 virus infection in Indonesia, July 2005-June 2006. *J. Infect. Dis.* 2007 Aug 15;196(4):522-7.

[82] Smith GJ, Naipospos TS, Nguyen TD, de Jong MD, Vijaykrishna D, Usman TB, Hassan SS, Nguyen TV, Dao TV, Bui NA, Leung YH, Cheung CL, Rayner JM, Zhang JX, Zhang LJ, Poon LL, Li KS, Nguyen VC, Hien TT, Farrar J, Webster RG, Chen H, Peiris JS, Guan Y. Evolution and adaptation of H5N1 influenza virus in avian and human hosts in Indonesia and Vietnam. *Virology.* 2006 Jul 5;350(2):258-68.

[83] Boltz DA, Douangngeun B, Sinthasak S, Phommachanh P, Rolston S, Chen H, Guan Y, Peiris JS, Smith JG, Webster RG. H5N1 influenza viruses in Lao People's Democratic Republic. *Emerg. Infect. Dis.* 2006 Oct;12(10):1593-5.

[84] Witt CJ, Malone JL. A veterinarian's experience of the spring 2004 avian influenza outbreak in Laos. *Lancet Infect. Dis.* 2005 Mar;5(3):143-5.

Chapter 4

Bird Flu in Western Countries

Bird Flu in Europe

A. Bird Flu in Turkey

Turkey is a country that lies in both Asia and Europe. This is the connecting site between the Eastern and Western world. The emergence of bird flu in Turkey was recently reported in the literature. The first avian influenza outbreak occurred on 5 October 2005 in northwest Turkey [1]. On 13 October 2005, the virus was confirmed as H5N1 in Weybridge CVL, AI-NDV Reference Laboratory [1]. Coven reported that the Turkish isolate had a direct relationship with recent Russian, Mongolian and Chinese isolates [1]. The second outbreak of AI in Turkey occurred on 26 December 2005 in Igdir, close to the Iranian and Armenian border [1]. The second outbreak was also due to H5N1 and it exhibited significant spreading potential within the eastern region of the country [1]. Human cases of influenza A H5N1 infection in eastern Turkey were first reported in December 2005-January 2006 [2] and there were continuous reports [3 – 7]. Oner et al. documented the epidemiologic, clinical, and radiologic features of all cases of confirmed H5N1 virus infection in patients who were admitted to the hospital in Turkey [8]. Oner et al. found that all of the patients had fever, and seven had clinical and radiologic evidence of pneumonia at presentation [8]. At present, there is no new human infection with H5N1 influenza virus in Turkey, but national measures and international support continue [9 - 16]. Akpinar and Saatci said that there was a substantial risk of either re-assortment of the virus, combination of avian and human influenza, or adaptation of the influenza virus to humans, and the situation in Turkey emphasized the importance of good surveillance and updated pandemic plans in all countries [17].

B. Bird Flu in Czech Republic

In order to determine the actual prevalence of avian influenza viruses in wild birds in the Czech Republic, extensive surveillance was carried out between January and April 2006 by Nagy et al. [18]. According to this work, highly pathogenic avian influenza virus subtype

H5N1 could be detected in Mute swans [18]. Surveillance of the disease is important for the Czech Republic. Indeed, a proposal for a plan of action for pandemic influenza caused by a new virus variant, the National Pandemic Plan of the Czech Republic (NPP-CR), was established since 2001 [19].

C. Bird Flu in Italy

Italy has faced bird flu problems many times. Many types of bird flu have ever been reported in Italy [20 - 28]. H5N1 is concern in Italy at present. The H5N1 virus was reported in swans in Italy [29]. In 2007, Cattoli et al. performed investigations of wild birds to assess the circulation of AI viruses in their natural reservoir [30]. According to this work, the isolates, belonging to eight different avian influenza virus subtype combinations (H10N4, H1N1, H4N6, H7N7, H7N4, H5N1, H5N2, and H5N3), were obtained from migratory Anseriformes [30]. The H5N1 infection has become a new disease under surveillance in Italy.

D. Bird Flu in the Netherlands

Similar to Italy, the Netherland has faced bird flu problems many times.
Many types of bird flu have been reported in the Netherlands [31 - 39]. H5N1 infection is not the main type of bird flu there [40 - 42].

E. Bird Flu in Romania

Epidemics of influenza have been sporadically reported in Romania for years [42 – 44]. Avian influenza H5N1 outbreaks in Romanian were reported in 2006 [45].

F. Bird Flu in Norway

The prevalence of influenza A virus infection, and the distribution of different subtypes of the virus, were studied in geese and ducks shot during ordinary hunting in 2005 in Norway [46]. Jonassen and Handeland reported that the H5N1 subtype was found in one mallard [46]. The other subtypes identified included H1N1, H2, H3N2, H3N8, H6N1, H6N2, H6N8, H8N4, H9N2, H11N9, and H12 in mallards; H3N2, H6N2, H6N8, and H9N2 in teals; and H6N2 in wigeons and common scoter [46].

G. Bird Flu in Austria

H5N1 infection can be seen in Austria. An interesting situation is the H5N1 infection in cats. Subclinical infection with avian influenza A H5N1 virus in cats in Austria was reported

[47-48]. Leschnick et al. said that avian influenza A virus subtype H5N1 was transmitted to domestic cats by close contact with infected birds [47].

H. Bird Flu In Bulgaria

Nota de Investigacón Bulgaria has a surveillance program for avian influenza to keep a close watch on the health of poultry, exotic birds, and wild birds [49]. Since October 2005, surveillance has become harder because of the situation in Romania and Turkey [49]. However, there is no report of H5N1 influenza virus.

I. Bird Flu in Spain

Spain is the origin of the most well-known influenza outbreak in humans in the past—, Spanish flu [50 - 57]. Notifiable bird flu had never been reported in Spain until July 2006, when a dead Great Crested Grebe (*Podiceps cristatus*) was found positive for the highly pathogenic H5N1 subtype as part of the active wild bird surveillance plan [58]. The current program of the Spanish Ministry of Agriculture, Fisheries, and Food (MAPA)'s strategic preventive plan against NAI can be divided into the following parts: identification of risk areas and at-risk wild bird species, increased biosecurity measures, early detection of infection with surveillance intensification and development of rapid diagnostic tests, and other policies, which include continuing education and training to ensure early detection of the disease [58].

However, avian H5N1 is not a present problem in Spain.

J. Bird Flu in Greece

Several wild migratory birds were confirmed to be infected with avian influenza A/H5N1 in Greece in February and March 2006 [59]. Several potential A/H5N1 human cases were recently identified in Greece; however, all were pseudo H5N1 infections [59]. The situation brought a lot attention from the general population in Greece. Marinos et al. attempted to assess the level of information among Greek students aged eight to 15 years, regarding avian influenza [60]. Marinos et al. found that the level of information about avian influenza among Greek students was satisfactory [60]. Marinos et al. noted that these findings, along with the potential for a future avian influenza pandemic, implied the need for intensified health education programs in Greek schools in order to deal with this serious public health problem [60].

K. Bird Flu in Portuguese

A program for the surveillance of influenza in Portugal has been in place for a long time [61]. It was noted that the prevalence of influenza A was associated with the occurrence of the highest number of influenza cases during December and January and the prevalence of influenza B with the occurrence of the highest number of influenza cases during February and March [61]. However, the presence of H5N1 infection is not a serious topic for the Portuguese.

L. Bird Flu in Denmark

The first introduction of highly pathogenic H5N1 avian influenza A viruses in wild and domestic birds in was reported in 2006 [62]. This was the first full genome characterization of HP H5N1 avian influenza A virus in the Nordic countries. Bragstad et al. reported that the Danish viruses had their origin in the wild bird strains from Qinghai in 2005 [62].

M. Bird Flu in Germany

H5N1 influenza virus can be seen in Germany [63]. In early 2006, the highly pathogenic avian influenza virus (HPAIV) H5N1 of the Asian lineage caused the death of wild aquatic birds in northern Germany [64]. During the recent outbreak of highly pathogenic avian influenza in Germany, mortality due to H5N1 highly pathogenic avian influenza was observed among mute and whooper swans as part of a rapid spread of this virus [65]. At necropsy, the most reliable lesions were multifocal hemorrhagic necrosis in the pancreas, pulmonary congestion and edema, and subepicardial hemorrhages [65].

In 2007, Klopfleisch et al. reported lesions and distribution of influenza virus antigen in three cats infected naturally with highly pathogenic avian influenza H5N1 A/swan/Germany/R65/06 [64]. Klopfleisch et al. showed that outdoor cats in areas affected by HPAIV in wild birds were at risk for lethal infection [64]. Analysis of the full-length sequences of all eight segments of the German wild-bird H5N1 highly pathogenic avian influenza virus index isolate, A/Cygnus cygnus/Germany/R65/2006, and an H5N1 isolate from a cat (A/cat/Germany/R606/2006) obtained during an outbreak in February 2006 revealed a very high similarity between these two sequences [66]. Multi-event imports of avian influenza virus A H5N1 into Bavaria, Germany were proposed [67]. Weber et al. said that reassortment events could be excluded in comparison with other 'Qinghai-like' H5N1 viruses. In addition, an H5N1 isolate originating from a single outbreak in poultry in Germany was found to be related closely to the H5N1 viruses circulating at that time in the wild-bird population [66]. According to a recent study by Greiner et al., a stochastic Monte-Carlo simulation was conducted which took into consideration (amongst others) the exposure and infection of chicken (broiler and layer), turkeys, ducks and geese; the probabilities of detection prior to slaughter; virus survival and contamination during slaughter; as well as during the cutting and preparation of meat in commercial plants and in private households, respectively [68]. The results show that the risk for the individual consumer is practically zero, as only up to 23 cases per year in Germany might occur [68]. Greiner et al. concluded that the finding of a low but non-negligible risk to the population should be a considerable point in the public health system of Germany [68].

N. Bird Flu in Russia

Bird flu in Russia is a big concern. A high diversity of highly pathogenic avian influenza H5N1 viruses that caused epizootic in Western Siberia was reported in 2005 [69]. Lipatov et al. recently studied influenza H5N1 viruses isolated from poultry in western Siberia and the European part of the Russian Federation during July 2005-February 2006 [70]. Lipatov et al. mentioned that phylogenetic analysis not only showed a close genetic relationship between the H5N1 strains isolated from poultry and wild migratory waterfowls but also suggested genetic reassortment among the analyzed isolates [70]. It is confirmed that H5N1 is an important problem in veterinarian science in Russia. The mass destruction of domestic birds was registered in July, 2005 in Novosibirsk region [71]. The phylogenetic analysis of hemagglutinin gene from the carcasses has shown that the isolated viruses were forming a cluster with strains isolated from birds during the outbreak of bird flu on lake Tsinghai (Qinghai) in China in 2005, in Japan in 2004, and also with H5N1 strains isolated from the person and birds in the countries of Southeast Asia during ipizootia in 2003-2004 [71]. However, for human infection, there has been no report. Karimova et al. also reported no detection of RNA and specific antibodies against influenza virus A H5N1 in human samples [72].

O. Bird Flu in the UK

H5N1 virus has been isolated in avians in the UK [63, 73]. Outbreaks of H5N1 influenza among avians in the UK were reported [73 – 74]. An integral part of the pandemic planning response in the UK was the creation in 2005 of the UK National H5 Laboratory Network, capable of rapidly and accurately identifying potential human H5N1 infections in all regions of the UK and the Republic of Ireland [75].

P. Bird Flu in Hungary

H5N1 has been seen in Hungary [76 - 79]. The relation between H5N1 in Hungary and UK was mentioned [76].

Bird Flu in America

A. Bird Flu in the USA [80 – 81]

Bird flu in the USA is of concern. There have been continuous reports of bird flu in the USA, but not the H5N1 types [82 - 84]. Under scrutiny are movements of birds and avian influenza from Asia into Alaska, the connection site to Asia [85]. However, there is no evidence of transferring of bird flu virus from Asia to Alaska [85]. In addition, Ortiz et al. reported that no evidence of H5N1 virus infection was found among American travelers suspected of having avian influenza A (H5N1) virus infection; none had direct contact with poultry, but 42% had evidence of human influenza A [86]. Although there are no reported cases, this disease is under strict control [87 - 90]. The use of Tamiflu as a prophylaxis agent in the event of a pandemic has been discussed [91 - 93]. Germann et al. said that the aggressive deployment of several million courses of influenza antiviral agents in a targeted prophylaxis strategy might contain a nascent outbreak, provided adequate contact tracing and distribution capacities existed [94].

Bird Flu in Canada

Although there have been bird flu outbreaks in the USA and Canada, there is no report of H5N1 influenza [95 – 102]. Similar to the USA, there are many disease control programs in place for a possible pandemic of H5N1 influenza in Canada.

References

[1]   Coven F. The Situation of Highly Pathogenic Avian Influenza (HPAI) Outbreaks in Turkey. *J. Vet. Med. B. Infect. Dis. Vet. Public Health.* 2006 Dec;53(s1):34.

[2]   Human cases of influenza A(H5N1) infection in eastern Turkey, December 2005-January 2006. *Wkly Epidemiol. Rec.* 2006 Oct 27;81(43):410-6.

[3]   More cases of avian influenza infection in humans and poultry in Turkey. *Euro Surveill.* 2006 Jan 12;11(1):E060112.1

[4]   Meijer A. Two fatal human infections with avian influenza H5, Turkey, January 2006. *Euro Surveill.* 2006 Jan 6;11(1):E060106.1.

[5]   Oner AF, Bay A, Arslan S, Akdeniz H, Sahin HA, Cesur Y, Epcacan S, Yilmaz N, Deger I, Kizilyildiz B, Karsen H, Ceyhan M. Avian influenza A (H5N1) infection in eastern Turkey in 2006. *N. Engl. J. Med.* 2006 Nov 23;355(21):2179-85.

[6]   Parry J.Z Children in Turkey die after contracting avian flu. *BMJ.* 2006 Jan 14;332(7533):67.

[7]   Enserink M. Avian influenza. More cases in Turkey, but no mutations found. *Science.* 2006 Jan 13;311(5758):161.

[8]   Influenza Team; International Outbreak Response Team in Turkey. No new human infections with A/H5N1 in Turkey but national measures and international support continue. *Euro Surveill.* 2006 Feb 2;11(2):E060202.2.

[9]   Outbreak news. Avian influenza, Turkey. *Wkly Epidemiol Rec.* 2006 Jan 13;81(2):13-5.

[10]   Outbreak news. Avian influenza, Turkey--update. *Wkly Epidemiol. Rec.* 2006 Jan 20;81(3):22-4.

[11]   Parry J. Turkey reports more cases as Asia prepares for bird flu. *BMJ.* 2006 Jan 21;332(7534):136.

[12]   Avian influenza. Amid mayhem in Turkey, experts see new chances for research. *Science.* 2006 Jan 20;311(5759):314-5.

[13]   Healy B. Let's talk Turkey. *US News World Rep.* 2006 Jan 23;140(3):64.

[14] OIE expresses concern about avian influenza in Turkey. *Vet. Rec.* 2006 Jan 14;158(2):34-5.

[15] Mayor S. Workers at UK turkey farm with symptoms of bird flu test negative for H5N1. *BMJ.* 2007 Feb 17;334(7589):335.

[16] Oncul O, Turhan V, Cavuslu S. H5N1 avian influenza: the Turkish dimension. *Lancet Infect Dis.* 2006 Apr;6(4):186-7.

[17] Akpinar E, Saatci E. Avian influenza in Turkey--will it influence health in all Europe? *Croat. Med. J.* 2006 Feb;47(1):7-15.

[18] Nagy A, Machova J, Hornickova J, Tomci M, Nagl I, Horyna B, Holko I. Highly pathogenic avian influenza virus subtype H5N1 in Mute swans in the Czech Republic. *Vet. Microbiol.* 2007 Feb 25;120(1-2):9-16.

[19] Polanecky V, Tumova B. A proposal of action plan for pandemic influenza caused by a new virus variant--the National Pandemic Plan of the Czech Republic (NPP-CR). *Cent. Eur. J. Public Health.* 2001 Nov;9(4):A-H.

[20] Mutinelli F, Capua I, Terregino C, Cattoli G. Clinical, gross, and microscopic findings in different avian species naturally infected during the H7N1 low- and high-pathogenicity avian influenza epidemics in Italy during 1999 and 2000. *Avian Dis.* 2003;47(3 Suppl):844-8.

[21] Mannelli A, Ferre N, Marangon S. Analysis of the 1999-2000 highly pathogenic avian influenza (H7N1) epidemic in the main poultry-production area in northern Italy. *Prev. Vet. Med.* 2006 Mar 16;73(4):273-85.

[22] Mulatti P, Kitron U, Mannelli A, Ferre N, Marangona S. Spatial analysis of the 1999-2000 highly pathogenic avian influenza (H7N1) epidemic in northern Italy. *Avian Dis.* 2007 Mar;51(1 Suppl):421-4.

[23] Di Trani L, Bedini B, Cordioli P, Muscillo M, Vignolo E, Moreno A, Tollis M. Molecular characterization of low pathogenicity H7N3 avian influenza viruses isolated in Italy. *Avian Dis.* 2004 Apr-Jun;48(2):376-83.

[24] Serena Beato M, Terregino C, Cattoli G, Capua I. Isolation and characterization of an H10N7 avian influenza virus from poultry carcasses smuggled from China into Italy. *Avian Pathol.* 2006 Oct;35(5):400-3.

[25] Rigoni M, Shinya K, Toffan A, Milani A, Bettini F, Kawaoka Y, Cattoli G, Capua I. Pneumo- and neurotropism of avian origin Italian highly pathogenic avian influenza H7N1 isolates in experimentally infected mice. *Virology.* 2007 Jul 20;364(1):28-35.

[26] Capua I, Marangon S. The use of vaccination to combat multiple introductions of Notifiable Avian Influenza viruses of the H5 and H7 subtypes between 2000 and 2006 in Italy. *Vaccine.* 2007 Jun 28;25(27):4987-95.

[27] Donatelli I, Campitelli L, Di Trani L, Puzelli S, Selli L, Fioretti A, Alexander DJ, Tollis M, Krauss S, Webster RG. Characterization of H5N2 influenza viruses from Italian poultry. *J. Gen. Virol.* 2001 Mar;82(Pt 3):623-30.

[28] Campitelli L, Fabiani C, Puzelli S, Fioretti A, Foni E, De Marco A, Krauss S, Webster RG, Donatelli I. H3N2 influenza viruses from domestic chickens in Italy: an increasing role for chickens in the ecology of influenza? *J. Gen. Virol.* 2002 Feb;83(Pt 2):413-20.

[29] Terregino C, Milani A, Capua I, Marino AM, Cavaliere N. Highly pathogenic avian influenza H5N1 subtype in mute swans in Italy. *Vet. Rec.* 2006 Apr 8;158(14):491.

[30] Cattoli G, Terregino C, Guberti V, De Nardi R, Drago A, Salviato A, Fassina S, Capua
      I. Influenza virus surveillance in wild birds in Italy: results of laboratory investigations
      in 2003-2005. *Avian Dis.* 2007 Mar;51(1 Suppl):414-6.

[31] Munster VJ, de Wit E, van Riel D, Beyer WE, Rimmelzwaan GF, Osterhaus AD,
      Kuiken T, Fouchier RA. The molecular basis of the pathogenicity of the Dutch highly
      pathogenic human influenza A H7N7 viruses. *J. Infect. Dis.* 2007 Jul 15;196(2):258-65.

[32] Elbers AR, Holtslag JB, Bouma A, Koch G. Within-flock mortality during the high-
      pathogenicity avian influenza (H7N7) epidemic in The Netherlands in 2003:
      implications for an early detection system. *Avian Dis.* 2007 Mar;51(1 Suppl):304-8.

[33] Bragstad K, Jorgensen PH, Handberg KJ, Fomsgaard A. Genome characterisation of
      the newly discovered avian influenza A H5N7 virus subtype combination. *Arch. Virol.*
      2007;152(3):585-93

[34] van der Goot JA, Koch G, de Jong MC, van Boven M. Quantification of the effect of
      vaccination on transmission of avian influenza (H7N7) in chickens. *Proc. Natl. Acad.
      Sci. U S A.* 2005 Dec 13;102(50):18141-6.

[35] Du Ry van Beest Holle M, Meijer A, Koopmans M, de Jager CM. Human-to-human
      transmission of avian influenza A/H7N7, The Netherlands, 2003. *Euro Surveill.* 2005
      Dec;10(12):264-8.

[36] Elbers AR, Koch G, Bouma A. Performance of clinical signs in poultry for the
      detection of outbreaks during the avian influenza A (H7N7) epidemic in The
      Netherlands in 2003. *Avian Pathol.* 2005 Jun;34(3):181-7.

[37] Thomas ME, Bouma A, Ekker HM, Fonken AJ, Stegeman JA, Nielen M. Risk factors
      for the introduction of high pathogenicity Avian Influenza virus into poultry farms
      during the epidemic in the Netherlands in 2003. *Prev. Vet. Med.* 2005 Jun 10;69(1-2):1-
      11.

[38] Bragstad K, Jorgensen PH, Handberg KJ, Mellergaard S, Corbet S, Fomsgaard A. New
      avian influenza A virus subtype combination H5N7 identified in Danish mallard ducks.
      Virus Res. 2005 May;109(2):181-90.

[39] Elbers AR, Fabri TH, de Vries TS, de Wit JJ, Pijpers A, Koch G. The highly
      pathogenic avian influenza A (H7N7) virus epidemic in The Netherlands in 2003--
      lessons learned from the first five outbreaks. *Avian Dis.* 2004 Sep;48(3):691-705.

[40] Timen A, van Vliet JA, Koopmans MP, van Steenbergen JE, Coutinho RA. Avian
      influenza H5NI in Europe: little risk as yet to health in the Netherlands. *Ned. Tijdschr.
      Geneeskd.* 2005 Nov 12;149(46):2547-9.

[41] Rahamat-Langendoen JC, van Vliet JA. Recent changes in the epidemiology of
      infectious diseases in the Netherlands: the report 'Status of infectious diseases in the
      Netherlands,' 2000-2005. *Ned. Tijdschr. Geneeskd.* 2007 Jun 16;151(24):1333-8.

[42] Magureanu E, Busuioc C, Ionescu V, Guguianu E, Stoicescu A, Horhogea G, Murgoci
      R, Coban V, Dobrescu A. Epidemiologic particularities of influenza in 1986 in a large
      urban centre of Romania. *Virologie.* 1987 Jul-Sep;38(3):195-204.

[43] Magureanu E, Busuioc C, Ionescu V, Guguianu E, Stoicescu A, Tisu A, Coban V,
      Stoianovici L, Dobrescu A. Epidemiological features of influenza in a large town of
      Romania during 1983. *Virologie.* 1985 Jan-Mar;36(1):15-22.

[44] Duca M, Handrache L, Morosanu V, Teodorovici G, Ivan A, Oana C, Zvoristeanu V, Groll M, Vieriu V, Mitroi I, et al. Influenza B in Moldavia (Romania) in the spring of 1984. *Rev. Med. Chir. Soc. Med. Nat. Iasi.* 1984 Oct-Dec;88(4):649-51.

[45] Avian influenza H5N1 outbreaks in Romanian and Danish poultry, and large H5N1 cluster in an Indonesian family. *Euro Surveill.* 2006 May 25;11(5):E060525.1

[46] Jonassen CM, Handeland K. Avian influenza virus screening in wild waterfowl in Norway, 2005. *Avian Dis.* 2007 Mar;51(1 Suppl):425-8.

[47] Leschnik M, Weikel J, Mostl K, Revilla-Fernandez S, Wodak E, Bago Z, Vanek E, Benetka V, Hess M, Thalhammer JG. Subclinical infection with avian influenza A (H5N1) virus in cats. *Emerg. Infect. Dis.* 2007 Feb;13(2):243-7.

[48] Burns K. Cats contract avian influenza virus. *J. Am. Vet. Med. Assoc.* 2006 Apr 15;228(8):1165-6.

[49] Goujgoulova G, Oreshkova N. Surveillance on avian influenza in Bulgaria. *Avian Dis.* 2007 Mar;51(1 Suppl):382-6.

[50] Webster RG. 1918 Spanish influenza: the secrets remain elusive. *Proc. Natl. Acad. Sci. U S A.* 1999 Feb 16;96(4):1164-6.

[51] Shortridge KF. The 1918 'Spanish' flu: pearls from swine? *Nat. Med.* 1999 Apr;5(4):384-5.

[52] Pennisi E. First genes isolated from the deadly 1918 flu virus. *Science.* 1997 Mar 21;275(5307):1739.

[53] Kaiser J. Virology. Resurrected influenza virus yields secrets of deadly 1918 pandemic. *Science.* 2005 Oct 7;310(5745):28-9.

[54] Shortridge KF. The 1918 'Spanish' flu: pearls from swine? *Nat. Med.* 1999 Apr;5(4):384-5.

[55] Taubenberger JK, Reid AH, Fanning TG. The 1918 influenza virus: A killer comes into view. *Virology.* 2000 Sep 1;274(2):241-5.

[56] Enserink M. Influenza. What came before 1918? Archaeovirologist offers a first glimpse. *Science.* 2006 Jun 23;312(5781):1725.

[57] Study of 1918 influenza pandemic virus provides information on origin and virulence mechanisms. *Euro Surveill.* 2005 Oct 20;10(10):E051020.1.

[58] Martinez M, Munoz MJ, De la Torre A, Martinez B, Iglesias I, Sanchez-Vizcaino JM. Risk assessment applied to Spain's prevention strategy against highly pathogenic avian influenza virus H5N1. *Avian Dis.* 2007 Mar;51(1 Suppl):507-11.

[59] Spala G, Panagiotopoulos T, Mavroidi N, Dedoukou X, Baka A, Tsonou P, Triantafyllou P, Mentis A, Kyriazopoulou V, Melidou A, Tsiodras S. A pseudo-outbreak of human A/H5N1 infections in Greece and its public health implications. *Euro Surveill.* 2006;11(11):263-7.

[60] Marinos G, Vasileiou I, Katsargyris A, Klonaris C, Georgiou C, Griniatsos J, Michail OP, Vlasis K, Giannopoulos A. Assessing the level of awareness of avian influenza among Greek students. *Rural Remote Health.* 2007 Jul-Sep;7(3):739.

[61] Falcao IM, de Andrade HR, Santos AS, Paixao MT, Falcao JM. Program for the surveillance of influenza in Portugal: results of the period 1990-1996. *J. Epidemiol. Community Health.* 1998 Apr;52 Suppl 1:39S-42S.

[62] Bragstad K, Jorgensen PH, Handberg K, Hammer AS, Kabell S, Fomsgaard A. First introduction of highly pathogenic H5N1 avian influenza A viruses in wild and domestic birds in Denmark, *Northern Europe*. Virol J. 2007 May 11;4:43.

[63] Avian influenza H5N1 detected in German poultry and a United Kingdom wild bird. *Euro Surveill*. 2006 Apr 6;11(4):E060406.1.

[64] Klopfleisch R, Wolf PU, Uhl W, Gerst S, Harder T, Starick E, Vahlenkamp TW, Mettenleiter TC, Teifke JP. Distribution of lesions and antigen of highly pathogenic avian influenza virus A/Swan/Germany/R65/06 (H5N1) in domestic cats after presumptive infection by wild birds. *Vet. Pathol.* 2007 May;44(3):261-8.

[65] Teifke JP, Klopfleisch R, Globig A, Starick E, Hoffmann B, Wolf PU, Beer M, Mettenleiter TC, Harder TC. Pathology of natural infections by H5N1 highly pathogenic avian influenza virus in mute (Cygnus olor) and whooper (Cygnus cygnus) swans. *Vet. Pathol.* 2007 Mar;44(2):137-43.

[66] Weber S, Harder T, Starick E, Beer M, Werner O, Hoffmann B, Mettenleiter TC, Mundt E. Molecular analysis of highly pathogenic avian influenza virus of subtype H5N1 isolated from wild birds and mammals in northern Germany. *J. Gen. Virol.* 2007 Feb;88(Pt 2):554-8.

[67] Rinder M, Lang V, Fuchs C, Hafner-Marx A, Bogner KH, Neubauer A, Buttner M, Rinder H. Genetic evidence for multi-event imports of avian influenza virus A (H5N1) into Bavaria, Germany. *J. Vet. Diagn. Invest.* 2007 May;19(3):279-82.

[68] Greiner M, Muller-Graf C, Hiller P, Schrader C, Gervelmeyer A, Ellerbroek L, Appel B. Expert opinion based modelling of the risk of human infection with H5N1 through the consumption of poultry meat in Germany. *Berl. Munch. Tierarztl. Wochenschr.* 2007 Mar-Apr;120(3-4):98-107.

[69] Evseenko VA, Zaykovskaya AV, Ternovoi VA, Durimanov AG, Zolotykh SI, Rassadkin YN, Lipatov AS, Webster RG, Shestopalov AM, Netesov SV, Drosdov IG, Onishchenko GG. Diversity of highly pathogenic avian influenza H5N1 viruses that caused epizootic in Western Siberia in 2005. *Dokl. Biol .Sci.* 2007 May-Jun;414:226-30.

[70] Lipatov AS, Evseenko VA, Yen HL, Zaykovskaya AV, Durimanov AG, Zolotykh SI, Netesov SV, Drozdov IG, Onishchenko GG, Webster RG, Shestopalov AM. Influenza (H5N1) viruses in poultry, Russian Federation, 2005-2006. *Emerg. Infect. Dis.* 2007 Apr;13(4):539-46.

[71] Onishchenko GG, Shestopalov AM, Ternovoi VA, Evseenko VA, Durymanov AG, Rassadkin IuN, Zaikovskaia AV, Zolotykh SI, Iurlov AK, Mikheev VN, Netesov SV, Drozdov IG. Study of highly pathogenic H5N1 influenza virus isolated from sick and dead birds in Western Siberia. *Zh. Mikrobiol. Epidemiol. Immunobiol.* 2006 Jul-Aug;(5):47-54.

[72] Karimova TV, Maliavina TA, Iakunina OI. Detection of RNA and specific antibodies against influenza virus A (H5N1) in human samples. *Zh. Mikrobiol. Epidemiol. Immunobiol.* 2006 Jul-Aug;(5):82-3.

[73] Outbreaks of highly pathogenic avian influenza (A/H5N1) in commercial poultry in Hungary and the UK--public health implications? *Euro Surveill*. 2007 Feb 15;12(2):E070215.3.

[74] Truscott J, Garske T, Chis-Ster I, Guitian J, Pfeiffer D, Snow L, Wilesmith J, Ferguson NM, Ghani AC. Control of a highly pathogenic H5N1 avian influenza outbreak in the GB poultry flock. *Proc. Biol. Sci.* 2007 Sep 22;274(1623):2287-95.

[75] Curran MD, Ellis JS, Wreghitt TG, Zambon MC. Establishment of a UK National Influenza H5 Laboratory Network. *J. Med. Microbiol.* 2007 Oct;56(Pt 10):1263-7.

[76] Mayor S. Link between H5N1 in UK and recent outbreaks in Hungary is investigated. *BMJ.* 2007 Feb 17;334(7589):335.

[77] Editorial team. Two outbreaks of H5N1 avian influenza in farm geese, Hungary, January 2007. *Euro Surveill.* 2007 Feb 15;12(2):E070215.2.

[78] Viruses responsible for avian influenza in Suffolk and Hungary "essentially identical". *Vet. Rec.* 2007 Feb 17;160(7):206.

[79] Influenza team the European Centre for Disease Prevention and Control. Outbreaks of highly pathogenic avian influenza (A/H5N1) in commercial poultry in Hungary and the UK--public health implications? *Euro Surveill.* 2007 Feb 15;12(2):E070215.3.

[80] Centers for Disease Control and Prevention (CDC). Update: influenza activity--United States and worldwide, May 20-September 15, 2007. *MMWR Morb. Mortal Wkly Rep.* 2007 Sep 28;56(38):1001-4.

[81] Centers for Disease Control and Prevention (CDC). Update: Influenza activity--United States and worldwide, 2006-07 season, and composition of the 2007-08 influenza vaccine. *MMWR Morb. Mortal Wkly Rep.* 2007 Aug 10;56(31):789-94.

[82] Lu H, Dunn PA, Wallner-Pendleton EA, Henzler DJ, Kradel DC, Liu J, Shaw DP, Miller P. Investigation of H7N2 avian influenza outbreaks in two broiler breeder flocks in Pennsylvania, 2001-02. *Avian Dis.* 2004 Jan-Mar;48(1):26-33.

[83] Dunn PA, Wallner-Pendleton EA, Lu H, Shaw DP, Kradel D, Henzler DJ, Miller P, Key DW, Ruano M, Davison S. Summary of the 2001-02 Pennsylvania H7N2 low pathogenicity avian influenza outbreak in meat type chickens. *Avian Dis.* 2003;47(3 Suppl):812-6.

[84] Henzler DJ, Kradel DC, Davison S, Ziegler AF, Singletary D, DeBok P, Castro AE, Lu H, Eckroade R, Swayne D, Lagoda W, Schmucker B, Nesselrodt A. Epidemiology, production losses, and control measures associated with an outbreak of avian influenza subtype H7N2 in Pennsylvania (1996-98). *Avian Dis.* 2003;47(3 Suppl):1022-36.

[85] Winker K, McCracken KG, Gibson DD, Pruett CL, Meier R, Huettmann F, Wege M, Kulikova IV, Zhuravlev YN, Perdue ML, Spackman E, Suarez DL, Swayne DE. Movements of birds and avian influenza from Asia into Alaska. *Emerg. Infect. Dis.* 2007 Apr;13(4):547-52.

[86] Ortiz JR, Wallis TR, Katz MA, Berman LS, Balish A, Lindstrom SE, Veguilla V, Teates KS, Katz JM, Klimov A, Uyeki TM. No evidence of avian influenza A (H5N1) among returning US travelers. *Emerg. Infect. Dis.* 2007 Feb;13(2):294-7.

[87] Myers J. Preparing for the worst. The real possibility that avian flu will hit the United States means all healthcare institutions need formal disaster recovery plans. *Healthc Inform.* 2006 Jul;23(7):44-5.

[88] Barlow BG. The potential for a pandemic? What the renal professional and patient need to know about avian flu. *Nephrol. News Issues.* 2006 Aug;20(9):42-6.

[89]   Center for Healthcare Environmental Management. Preparing for avian flu. *Healthc Hazard Manage Monit.* 2006 Aug;19(12):1-8.

[90]   Mika M. National plan for pandemic flu unveiled. *JAMA.* 2006 Jun 21;295(23):2707-8.

[91]   Ludwig G. Avian flu: nothing to sneeze at. *JEMS.* 2006 Jun;31(6):20.

[92]   Centers for Disease Control and Prevention. Pandemic influenza update. *J. Med. Assoc. Ga.* 2005;94(3-4):26-7.

[93]   O'Malley P. Bird flu pandemic and Tamiflu: implications for the clinical nurse specialist. *Clin. Nurse Spec.* 2006 Mar-Apr;20(2):65-7.

[94]   Schwartz ND. The Tamiflu tug of war. *Fortune.* 2005 Nov 14;152(10):33-4.

[95]   Matsumoto K. Flu epidemic: shots, new treatments available. *AIDS Treat News.* 2000 Jan 21;(No 335):2-4.

[96]   Germann TC, Kadau K, Longini IM Jr, Macken CA. Mitigation strategies for pandemic influenza in the United States. *Proc. Natl. Acad.Sci. U S A.* 2006 Apr 11;103(15):5935-40.

[97]   Reyes F, Aziz S, Macey JF, Winchester B, Zabchuk P, Wootton S, Huston P, Tam TW. Influenza in Canada: 2006-2007 season update. *Can. Commun. Dis. Rep.* 2007 May 1;33(9):85-92.

[98]   Senne DA. Avian influenza in North and South America, 2002-2005. *Avian Dis.* 2007 Mar;51(1 Suppl):167-73.

[99]   Bowes BA. After the outbreak: how the British Columbia commercial poultry industry recovered after H7N3 HPAI. *Avian Dis.* 2007 Mar;51(1 Suppl):313-6.

[100] Reyes F, Macey JF, Aziz S, Li Y, Watkins K, Winchester B, Zabchuck P, Zheng H, Huston P, Tam TW, Hatchette T. Influenza in Canada: 2005-2006 season. *Can. Commun. Dis. Rep.* 2007 Feb 1;33(3):21-41.

[101] MacDougall H. Toronto's Health Department in action: influenza in 1918 and SARS in 2003. *J. Hist. Med. Allied Sci.* 2007 Jan;62(1):56-89.

[102] Influenza in Canada--2004-2005 season. *Can. Commun. Dis. Rep.* 2006 Mar 15;32(6):57-74.

[103] Influenza in Canada: 2005-2006 season update. *Can. Commun. Dis. Rep.* 2006 Feb 15;32(4):38-43.

[104] The epidemiology of influenza in children hospitalized in Canada, 2004-2005, in Immunization Monitoring Program Active (IMPACT) centres. *Can. Commun Dis. Rep.* 2006 Apr 1;32(7):77-86.

Chapter 5

Clinical Manifestations of Human Bird Flu Infection

Common History of Human H5N1 Infected Cases

Human infection of H5N1 is a new emerging infectious disease. Most infected cases have a history of contact with sick avians [1 – 4]. The patients usually presented with fever and respiratory symptoms [1 – 2]. Thorson et al. performed research to analyze the association between flulike illness, defined as cough and fever, and exposure to sick or dead poultry [3]. Thorson et al. found that epidemiological data were consistent with transmission of mild, highly pathogenic avian influenza to humans and suggested that transmission could be more common than anticipated, though close contact seemed required [3]. They noted that further microbiological studies were needed to validate these findings [3]. In this chapter, the details of clinical manifestation of human bird flu infection will be summarized and presented. To evaluate risk factors for human infection with influenza A subtype H5N1, Dinh et al. performed a matched case-control study in Vietnam [5]. They noted that factors not significantly associated with infection were raising healthy poultry, preparing healthy poultry for consumption, and exposure to persons with an acute respiratory illness [5]. Vong et al. conducted a retrospective survey of poultry deaths and a seroepidemiologic investigation in a Cambodian village where a 28-year-old man was infected with H5N1 virus in March 2005 [6]. Despite frequent, direct contact with poultry suspected of having H5N1 virus infection, none of 351 participants from 93 households had neutralizing antibodies to H5N1 [6]. Vong et al. said that H5N1 virus transmission from poultry to humans remained low in this setting and set a question for other possible modes of transmission of H5N1 [6]. In 2005, Ungchusak et al. investigated possible person-to-person transmission in a family cluster of the disease in Thailand [7]. The index patient became ill three to four days after her last exposure to dying household chickens [7]. Her mother came from a far-away city to care for her in the hospital, had no recognized exposure to poultry, and died from pneumonia [7]. The aunt also provided unprotected nursing care; she had fever five days after the mother first had fever, followed by pneumonia seven days later [7]. Of interest, autopsy tissue from the mother and nasopharyngeal and throat swabs from the aunt were positive for H5N1 by reverse transcriptase polymerase chain reaction [7]. Ungchusak et al. concluded that disease in the mother and aunt probably resulted from person-to-person transmission of this deadly avian influenza virus during unprotected exposure to the critically ill index patient [7].

Fever in Bird Flu Infection

Indeed, fever is a common manifestation and nonspecific for many infections. However, there are some interesting reports concerning fever in H5N1 infection. It should be noted that H5N1 viruses can hyper-induce cytokines (tumor necrosis factor [TNF] alpha, interferon beta) and chemokines (IP10, MIP1alpha, MCP) in *in vitro* cultures of primary human macrophages and these can be the cause of fever appearance [8]. Seo et al. said that pigs infected with recombinant human H1N1 influenza virus that carried the H5N1 NS gene experienced significantly greater and more prolonged viremia, fever, and weight loss than did pigs infected with wild-type human H1N1 influenza virus [9]. Seo et al. noted that these effects required the presence of glutamic acid at position 92 of the NS1 molecule [9 - 10]. They concluded that these findings might explain the mechanism of the high virulence of H5N1 influenza viruses in humans and provide insight into the virulence of 1918 Spanish influenza [9]. Banning said that influenza could begin suddenly and was accompanied by fever, chills, aches, pains, headaches, fatigue, coughing and generalized weakness that can last up to 14 days [11].

Respiratory Manifestation of Bird Flu Infection

The symptoms of avian influenza range from typical influenza symptoms - fever, cough, sore throat and muscle ache - to eye infection, pneumonia, respiratory distress and other, sometimes fatal, complications [12]. Severe complications arising from pandemic influenza or the highly pathogenic avian H5N1 viruses are often associated with rapid, massive inflammatory cell infiltration, acute respiratory distress, reactive hemophagocytosis, and multiple organ involvement [13]. Angelava et al. said that initial symptoms of the H5N1 influenza are: fever greater than 38 degrees Celsius, mild cold, cough and shortness of breath, viral pneumonia (in most patients), later secondary bacterial infection, mild to severe respiratory distress, diarrhea, vomiting and abdominal pain [12]. Angela et al. also mentioned that sometimes gastrointestinal disorder begins a week earlier than respiratory symptoms [12]. The patients usually show clinical and radiological signs of pneumonia with radiological alterations that include diffuse infiltrates and lobar or segmentary consolidations on air bronchogram [12]. Effects of microbial aerosol application on the pathogenesis and clinical pictures of aerosol infection at the site are well described [13]. A relationship was revealed among the fractional-dispersive composition of the microbial aerosol, the portal of infection, and the clinico-pathogenetic peculiarities of the course of the disease [14]. Influenza is a very small viral particle and classified as highly-dispersive aerosol that can lead to the appearance of primary pneumonia [14]. Apoptosis can be observed in alveolar epithelial cells, which is the major target cell type for viral replication [14]. Uiprasertkul said that apoptosis might play a major role in the pathogenesis of H5N1 influenza virus in humans by destroying alveolar epithelial cells [15]. Uiprasertkul also mentioned that this pathogenesis causes pneumonia and destroys leukocytes, leading to leukopenia, which is a prominent clinical feature of influenza H5N1 virus in humans [5]. La Gruta et al. noted that various effector arms of the immune system could act deleteriously to initiate or exacerbate pathological damage in this viral pneumonia [13]. Biologically active interferon-alpha, tumor necrosis factor-alpha (TNF-alpha), and interleukin-1 (IL-1) were detected in bronchoalveolar lavage (BAL) fluids of deprived pigs inoculated with H1N1 influenza virus by Van Reeth et al. [16]. This study is the first demonstration of TNF-alpha and IL-1 in BAL fluids of a natural influenza virus host [16]. It documents that pigs may be a highly valuable experimental model in human influenza virus pneumonia [16]. The role of IL-18 in the development of the host defence system against influenza virus infection was investigated by Liu et al. in 2004 [17]. Liu et al. reported that local immune responses in the lung such as specific cytotoxic T lymphocyte and antibody production were induced upon influenza virus infection [17]. These results indicate that IL-18 is involved in controlling influenza virus replication in the lung, especially at an early stage of infection, through activation of the innate immune mechanisms such as IFN and NK cells [17]. This mechanism is also believed to be an important pathogenesis for H5N1 pneumonia [18]. Peper and Van Campen reported another animal model study to support this proposal. They reported that the severity of gross and histologic lung lesions positively correlated with the peak bronchoalveolar TNF alpha levels and was ameliorated with anti-TNF alpha treatment [18]. They suggested that TNF alpha was a mediator of pulmonary inflammation during influenza A viral pneumonia, but might not play a significant anti-viral role in influenza pneumonia [18]. Savitskii et al. noted that the activity of natural killers in uncomplicated influenza in the acute period of the disease was higher, and in patients with influenza complicated by pneumonia lower than in normal subjects [19].

Chest X ray remains the most convenient and accessible imaging modality for diagnosis of H5N1 pneumonia. Qureshi et al. said that several studies had shown that most radiographs are abnormal at the time of presentation with multifocal consolidation the most common radiographic finding [20]. They noted that pleural effusions and cavitation could also develop during the course of disease [20]. They proposed that consolidation that involved equal or more than four zones on presentation or at day seven after the onset of symptoms and subsequent development of acute respiratory distress syndrome were generally associated with an adverse outcome [20]. Bay et al. reported that the major radiologic abnormalities were extensive pneumonic infiltration with segmental and multifocal distribution, mostly located in lower zones of the lung [21]. Bay et al. concluded that avian flu might be presented as rapidly progressive pneumonia [21]. They noted that chest X ray had an important role in diagnosis and should be obtained daily because of rapid change of the findings that may necessitate prompt action [21]. For computerized tomogram, Qureshi et al. said that persistent ground glass attenuation and segmental consolidation were common in the convalescent stage [20]. Additional mild fibrotic features included pseudocavitation, pneumatocoele formation, lymphadenopathy, and centrilobular nodules [20]. Indeed, these findings are characteristic of fulminant influenza pneumonia [22].

The first case of H5N1 avian influenza infection in a human with complications of adult respiratory distress syndrome (ARDS) and Reye's syndrome was reported in 1999 [23]. ARDS is common in fatal human H5N1 infected cases [24]. Carter proposed that steroid might be useful for severe acquired respiratory syndromes and avian influenza [25]. Carter said that the steroid usage prevented the resultant hypercytokinaemia from developing if the patient did not seek timely medical assistance [25].

Ocular Manifestation of Bird Flu Infection

Ocular disturbance can be seen in bird flu infection. Conjunctivitis is a common clinical presentation of infected patients. The H7N7 is well documented for conjunctivitis [26 - 27]. A highly pathogenic avian influenza A virus of subtype H7N7, closely related to low pathogenic virus isolates obtained from wild ducks, was isolated from chickens [26]. Fouchier et al. said that avian influenza A virus (H7N7) was associated with human conjunctivitis and a fatal case of acute respiratory distress syndrome [26]. They reported that from 78 to 89 cases of H7N7 bird flu infection presented with conjunctivitis [26]. For H7N3, conjunctivitis is also mentioned. An outbreak of low pathogenicity H7N3 avian influenza in the UK, including an associated case of human conjunctivitis was recently reported in 2006 in the UK [28]. A similar outbreak was also reported in British Columbia in 2004 [29]. The main symptoms of H7N3 include conjunctivitis and mild influenza-like illness. For H5N1 influenza infection, conjunctivitis is not well described in human infection but it is well described in chickens with H5N1 influenza infection [30].

Gastrointestinal Manifestation of Bird Flu Infection

The gastrointestinal tract is a highly-affected area in infected avians. Gastrointestinal manifestations in infected humans can also be seen. There have been some reports of diarrhea in severe bird flu infection [31]. Poovorawan recently proposed that diarrhea was an important presentation of bird flu and could imply a poor prognosis [32]. Wiwanitkit attempted to assess the magnitude of diarrhea among Thai infected cases and its correlation with infection outcome [33]. According to this study, the prevalence of diarrheal presentation was high, similar to a recent study in Vietnam (approximately 70 %) [1]. Of interest, diarrhea usually correlated with high fatality in H5N1 influenza infection [34]. For example, Witayathawornwong reported a fatal case of H5N1 infection in Thailand [34]. In this case, ARDS was documented from the time of admission, mechanical ventilation was introduced without improvement, and she had multiple episodes of diarrhea for two days before death [34]. Zhang et al. reported another case of H5N1 in China [35]. The initial symptoms in this fatal case included high fever with influenza-like symptoms, and then cough and purulent sputum mixed with blood appeared [35]. The clinical situation deteriorated progressively with occurrence of diarrhea and dyspnea [35]. Wiwanitkit therefore concluded that diarrheal presentation had a correlation with poor outcome among infected Thai subjects [33].

Another important point to be addressed is that diarrhea can be an adverse effect of antiviral drugs. Acute hemorrhagic colitis induced by the neuraminidase inhibitor oseltamivir is documented. Yoneda et al. reported a 23-year-old woman with lower abdominal pain, diarrhea and bloody stool who was admitted and given a diagnosis of influenza B and treated by oseltamivir [36]. After treatment, this patient developed bloody diarrhea due to acute hemorrhagic colitis [36]. In addition to diarrhea, vomiting and abdominal pain are two other common gastrointestinal manifestations in bird flu infection [37]. After a typical H1N1 influenza illness, the patient can sometimes develop hematemesis of varying severity. However, this has never been documented in H5N1 infection. However, there was a report on H3N2 avian flu infection [38]. The patient presented with acute symptoms of abdominal pain, vomiting, and syncope in the hour preceding the shock [38]. During both episodes, necessary management included aggressive intravenous fluid rehydration, mechanical ventilation, and use of inotropes/vasopressors [38]. Systemic capillary leak syndrome presenting as recurrent shock was also described in this case [38].

Concerning hepatic manifestation of bird flu infection, there have been no reports in this area. Here, the author performs a mini-study in order to document the impact of bird flu infection on the level of transaminase enzymes among reported Thai patients. A literature review on the papers concerning human bird flu in Thailand was performed. The author performed the literature review of human bird flu infection reports in Thailand from the databases of the published works cited in the *Index Medicus* and *Science Citation Index*. The author also reviewed the published works in all 256 local Thai journals, which is not included in the international citation index, for reports of human bird flu infection in Thailand. The reports that contained no complete data were excluded from further analysis. According to this review, there are six reports [39 – 44] covering 12 Thai patients with confirmed diagnosis of bird flu. However, the complete data for levels of transaminase enzymes were available on only six patients. The reported SGOT ranges from 120 U/L to 790 U/L with average value equal to 367.8 ± 80.2 U/L (median = 280.0 U/L). The reported SGPT ranges from 43 U/L to 150 U/L with average value equal to 80.2 ± 46.4 U/L (median = 52.0 U/L). Here, the elevation of the transaminase enzymes, especially extremely elevated levels of SGOT, can be seen. These findings agree with the report on the outbreak in Hong Kong that liver dysfunction was common [45]. This implies that hepatitis might be an important manifestation of human bird flu infection. The H5N1 virus itself might be part of the cause of liver pathology.

Neurological Manifestation of Bird Flu Infection

Infections caused by influenza viruses can be very serious and may even lead to death resulting from the post-infectious complications [46]. The most commonly-occurring complications are pneumonia, bronchitis, bronchiolitis, myocarditis and otitis media [46]. The other group is neurological post-influenza complications, including dementia, epileptic disorders, cerebrovascular disease, febrile convulsions, toxic encephalopathy, encephalitis, meningitis, subarachnoid hemorrhages, psychosis or increase in the number of cases of Parkinson's disease [46]. Neurological manifestations of bird flu infection is of concern in avian infections. They may be classified into several subtypes according to the clinical symptoms and laboratory data [47]. Unfortunately, pathogenesis of encephalopathy and encephalitis after infection with viruses of influenza is still unclear [48]. This problem seems very important because most neurological cases, especially for encephalopathy and encephalitis after influenza , are seen in children and adolescents, who have not yet complete immunological protecting mechanisms [48]. Togashi et al. studied the epidemiology of influenza-associated encephalitis-encephalopathy in Hokkaido, the northernmost island of Japan [49]. According to this study, most affected patients became comatose with or without convulsions within a few days of the onset of fever [49]. Togashi et al. said that brain CT abnormalities had a poor prognosis [49]. Togashi et al. concluded that it appeared urgent to promote vaccination against influenza in young children to prevent these devastating disease conditions [49]. Rowe et al. said that intranasal infection of mice with HK/483, but not HK/486, resulted in viral spread to the brain, neurologic signs, and death; however, HK/486 was able to replicate in the brain and induce lethal disease following direct intracerebral inoculation [50]. In human infection, Govorkova et al. said that the severity of disease was associated with a broad tissue tropism and high virus titers in multiple organs, including the brain [51]. In some fatal human cases, H5N1 can be isolated [31]. Seizures and coma are common among those cases [31].

Ear Manifestations in Bird Flu Infection

As previously mentioned, otitis can be seen as complication of influenza. Pappas and Owen Hendley said that yearly administration of the influenza vaccine and/or treatment of influenza with an antiviral (oseltamivir) could significantly decrease the incidence of acute otitis media during influenza season [52]. Major pathologies observed in the ear include a general inflammatory cell infiltration, vacuolation and other degeneration of ciliated cells, and vascular damage and increased vascular permeability [53]. Regeneration of cilia or ciliated cells followed the degeneration, which included an increased number of basal cells and new formed centrioles [53]. Sugiura et al. said that viral infection could evoke mucociliary dysfunction of the tubotympanum and create an increased susceptibility to bacteria; therefore, viral infection could enhance the bacterial process in the tubotympanum [53]. Tong et al. also suggested a synergic effects of influenza A virus and *Streptococcus pneumoniae* on the changes of the carbohydrate moieties in the eustatian tube epithelium [54]. Tong et al. also indicated that influenza A virus promoted a significant increase in nasopharyngeal colonization by *Streptococcus pneumoniae*, an increased incidence and severity of otitis media, and a sustained presence of *Streptococcus pneumoniae* in the effusions [55]. However, the correlation between otitis and bird flu infection is rarely reported.

Nephrological Manifestations of Bird Flu Infection

Nephrological manifestations of bird flu infection can be seen. Renal insufficiency [56] and increased blood creatinine level [57] can be detected. It is postulated that, in fatal human infections with this avian subtype, the initial virus replication in the respiratory tract triggers hypercytokinemia complicated by other organ involvement [56]. Renal involvement of bird flu infection has been reported. To et al. recently reported the autopsy findings of acute renal failure (ARF) in fatal human bird flu infection [58]. However, the pathogenesis underlying the renal involvement in still not clear. Wiwanitkit said that although the fatality rate in patients with renal insufficiency was higher than in those without, there was no significant correlation between the presence of renal insufficiency and the development of ARDS or fatality [56].

Cardiovascular Manifestations of Bird Flu Infection

Cardiovascular manifestations of bird flu infection have been reported. Wiwanitkit proposed that hypertension can be seen in bird flu infection [59]. Indeed, cardiovascular complication is well documented in general influenza infection. Podolec and Kopec proposed that vaccination can decrease cardiovascular complications of infection [60]. In infected avian, H5N1 virus can be detected in heart tissue [61]. Antarasena et al. demonstrated the usefulness of the cardiac tissue from infected chickens, quail, and ducks for diagnosis [61]. Wiwanitkit also reported that cardiogenic shock was common in fatal human H5N1 infected cases [62].

Joint Manifestations of Bird Flu Infection

Joint pain is a common complaint in patients with influenza [63]. Fever, myalgia and arthralgia are common in general influenza. One explanation for these symptoms may be that they are due to extra-respiratory transmission of virus by viremia [64]. However, there is no report on bird flu infection. Further study of this area is recommended.

Hematological Manifestations of Bird Flu Infection

Hematological manifestations of bird flu infection are well documented. Wiwanitkit noted that anemia [65] as well as thrombocytopenia [66] could be found in human H5N1 infected cases. Wiwanitkit concluded that the main hematologic manifestation of H5N1 infection is lymphopenia with decreased lymphocyte/neutrophil ratio. Anemia can also be observed in this infection [67]. The effects of this infection on platelets are still controversial [67]. More details on hematological laboratory changes will be discussed on the chapter on pathology of bird flu.

References

[1] Tran TH, Nguyen TL, Nguyen TD, Luong TS, Pham PM, Nguyen VC, Pham TS, Vo CD, Le TQ, Ngo TT, Dao BK, Le PP, Nguyen TT, Hoang TL, Cao VT, Le TG, Nguyen DT, Le HN, Nguyen KT, Le HS, Le VT, Christiane D, Tran TT, Menno de J, Schultsz C, Cheng P, Lim W, Horby P, Farrar J; World Health Organization International Avian Influenza Investigative Team. Avian influenza A (H5N1) in 10 patients in Vietnam. *N. Engl. J. Med.* 2004 Mar 18;350(12):1179-88.

[2] Chotpitayasunondh T, Ungchusak K, Hanshaoworakul W, Chunsuthiwat S, Sawanpanyalert P, Kijphati R, Lochindarat S, Srisan P, Suwan P, Osotthanakorn Y, Anantasetagoon T, Kanjanawasri S, Tanupattarachai S, Weerakul J, Chaiwirattana R, Maneerattanaporn M, Poolsavathitikool R, Chokephaibulkit K, Apisarnthanarak A, Dowell SF. Human disease from influenza A (H5N1), Thailand, 2004. *Emerg. Infect. Dis.* 2005 Feb;11(2):201-9.

[3] Thorson A, Petzold M, Nguyen TK, Ekdahl K. Is exposure to sick or dead poultry associated with flulike illness?: a population-based study from a rural area in Vietnam with outbreaks of highly pathogenic avian influenza. *Arch. Intern. Med.* 2006 Jan 9;166(1):119-23.

[4] Groome PA, Richardson H. Flulike illness and exposure to sick or dead poultry. *Arch. Intern. Med.* 2006 Jul 10;166(13):1420-1.

[5] Dinh PN, Long HT, Tien NT, Hien NT, Mai le TQ, Phong le H, Tuan le V, Van Tan H, Nguyen NB, Van Tu P, Phuong NT; World Health Organization/Global Outbreak Alert and Response Network Avian Influenza Investigation Team in Vietnam. Risk factors for human infection with avian influenza A H5N1, Vietnam, 2004. *Emerg. Infect. Dis.* 2006 Dec;12(12):1841-7.

[6] Vong S, Coghlan B, Mardy S, Holl D, Seng H, Ly S, Miller MJ, Buchy P, Froehlich Y, Dufourcq JB, Uyeki TM, Lim W, Sok T. Low frequency of poultry-to-human H5N1 virus transmission, southern Cambodia, 2005. *Emerg. Infect. Dis.* 2006 Oct;12(10):1542-7.

[7] Ungchusak K, Auewarakul P, Dowell SF, Kitphati R, Auwanit W, Puthavathana P, Uiprasertkul M, Boonnak K, Pittayawonganon C, Cox NJ, Zaki SR, Thawatsupha P, Chittaganpitch M, Khontong R, Simmerman JM, Chunsutthiwat S. Probable person-to-person transmission of avian influenza A (H5N1). *N. Engl. J. Med.* 2005 Jan 27;352(4):333-40.

[8] Seo SH, Hoffmann E, Webster RG. The NS1 gene of H5N1 influenza viruses circumvents the host anti-viral cytokine responses. *Virus Res.* 2004 Jul;103(1-2):107-13.

[9] Seo SH, Hoffmann E, Webster RG. Lethal H5N1 influenza viruses escape host anti-viral cytokine responses. *Nat. Med.* 2002 Sep;8(9):950-4.

[10] Banning M. Influenza: incidence, symptoms and treatment. *Br J Nurs.* 2005 Dec 8-2006 Jan 11;14(22):1192-7.

[11] Viejo Bañuelos JL Respiratory manifestations of avian influenza. *Arch. Bronconeumol.* 2006 Dec;42(Supl.2):12-18.

[12] Angelava NA, Angelava AV. Epidemiology, clinical picture, prevention and treatment of Avian influenza. *Georgian Med. News.* 2006 Feb;(131):69-76.

[13] La Gruta NL, Kedzierska K, Stambas J, Doherty PC. A question of self-preservation: immunopathology in influenza virus infection. *Immunol Cell Biol.* 2007 Feb-Mar;85(2):85-92

[14] Gapochko KG. Effect of the site of microbial aerosol application on the pathogenesis and clinical picture of aerosol infection. *Zh. Mikrobiol. Epidemiol. Immunobiol.* 1976 Aug;(8):78-83.

[15] Uiprasertkul M. Apoptosis and Pathogenesis of Avian Influenza A (H5N1) Virus in Humans. *Emerg. Infect. Dis.* 2007 May;13(5):708-12.

[16] Van Reeth K, Nauwynck H, Pensaert M. Bronchoalveolar interferon-alpha, tumor necrosis factor-alpha, interleukin-1, and inflammation during acute influenza in pigs: a possible model for humans? *J. Infect. Dis.* 1998 Apr;177(4):1076-9.

[17] Liu B, Mori I, Hossain MJ, Dong L, Takeda K, Kimura Y. Interleukin-18 improves the early defence system against influenza virus infection by augmenting natural killer cell-mediated cytotoxicity. *J. Gen. Virol.* 2004 Feb;85(Pt 2):423-8.

[18] Peper RL, Van Campen H. Tumor necrosis factor as a mediator of inflammation in influenza A viral pneumonia. *Microb. Pathog.* 1995 Sep;19(3):175-83.

[19] Savitskii GI, Grishchenko SV, Krylov VF, Kolobukhina LV, Kniazeva LD. Natural killer activity in influenza patients. *Vopr. Virusol.* 1988 May-Jun;33(3):290-2.

[20] Qureshi NR, Hien TT, Farrar J, Gleeson FV. The radiologic manifestations of H5N1 avian influenza. *J. Thorac. Imaging.* 2006 Nov;21(4):259-64.

[21] Bay A, Etlik O, Oner AF, Unal O, Arslan H, Bora A, Davran R, Yuca SA, Dogan M. Radiological and clinical course of pneumonia in patients with avian influenza H5N1. *Eur. J. Radiol.* 2007 Feb;61(2):245-50.

[22] Berdal JE, Smith-Erichsen N. Fulminant influenza pneumonia. *Tidsskr. Nor. Laegeforen.* 2000 Jan 30;120(3):312-4.

[23] Ku AS, Chan LT. The first case of H5N1 avian influenza infection in a human with complications of adult respiratory distress syndrome and Reye's syndrome. *J. Paediatr. Child Health.* 1999 Apr;35(2):207-9.

[24] Arabi Y, Gomersall CD, Ahmed QA, Boynton BR, Memish ZA. The critically ill avian influenza A (H5N1) patient. *Crit. Care Med.* 2007 May;35(5):1397-403.

[25] Carter MJ. A rationale for using steroids in the treatment of severe cases of H5N1 avian influenza. *J. Med. Microbiol.* 2007 Jul;56(Pt 7):875-83.

[26] Fouchier RA, Schneeberger PM, Rozendaal FW, Broekman JM, Kemink SA, Munster V, Kuiken T, Rimmelzwaan GF, Schutten M, Van Doornum GJ, Koch G, Bosman A, Koopmans M, Osterhaus AD. Avian influenza A virus (H7N7) associated with human conjunctivitis and a fatal case of acute respiratory distress syndrome. *Proc. Natl. Acad. Sci. U S A.* 2004 Feb 3;101(5):1356-61.

[27] Munster VJ, de Wit E, van Riel D, Beyer WE, Rimmelzwaan GF, Osterhaus AD, Kuiken T, Fouchier RA. The molecular basis of the pathogenicity of the Dutch highly pathogenic human influenza A H7N7 viruses. *J. Infect. Dis.* 2007 Jul 15;196(2):258-65.

[28] Nguyen-Van-Tam JS, Nair P, Acheson P, Baker A, Barker M, Bracebridge S, Croft J, Ellis J, Gelletlie R, Gent N, Ibbotson S, Joseph C, Mahgoub H, Monk P, Reghitt TW,

Sundkvist T, Sellwood C, Simpson J, Smith J, Watson JM, Zambon M, Lightfoot N; Incident Response Team. Outbreak of low pathogenicity H7N3 avian influenza in UK, including associated case of human conjunctivitis. *Euro Surveill.* 2006 May 4;11(5):E060504.2.

[29] Tweed SA, Skowronski DM, David ST, Larder A, Petric M, Lees W, Li Y, Katz J, Krajden M, Tellier R, Halpert C, Hirst M, Astell C, Lawrence D, Mak A. Human illness from avian influenza H7N3, British Columbia. *Emerg. Infect. Dis.* 2004 Dec;10(12):2196-9.

[30] Vascellari M, Granato A, Trevisan L, Basilicata L, Toffan A, Milani A, Mutinelli F. Pathologic Findings of Highly Pathogenic Avian Influenza Virus A/Duck/Vietnam/12/05 (H5N1) in Experimentally Infected Pekin Ducks, Based on Immunohistochemistry and In Situ Hybridization. *Vet. Pathol.* 2007 Sep;44(5):635-42.

[31] de Jong MD, Bach VC, Phan TQ, Vo MH, Tran TT, Nguyen BH, Beld M, Le TP, Truong HK, Nguyen VV, Tran TH, Do QH, Farrar J. Fatal avian influenza A (H5N1) in a child presenting with diarrhea followed by coma. *N. Engl. J. Med.* 2005;352:686–91.

[32] Poovorawan Y. Avian influenza H51N1: the changing situation. *J. Med. Tech. Assoc. Thai.* 2005;33 (suppl 1) :26–32.

[33] Wiwanitkit V. Diarrhoea as a presentation of bird flu infection: a summary on its correlation to outcome in Thai cases. *Gut.* 2005 Oct;54(10):1506.

[34] Witayathawornwong P. Avian influenza A (H5N1) infection in a child. Southeast Asian *J. Trop. Med. Public Health.* 2006 Jul;37(4):684-9.

[35] Zhang W, Wen LY, Lu M, Xiong Y, Qian KJ, Deng AH, Guo LS, Xiao ZK, Zhao XS, Duan SM, Xie ZG, Gao ZF, Li M, Shao HQ, Wang GG, Liu DW, Gao ZC. Clinical characteristic analysis of the first human case infected by influenza A (H5N1) in Jiangxi Province. *Zhonghua Jie He He Hu Xi Za Zhi.* 2006 May;29(5):300-6.

[36] Yoneda S, Kobayashi Y, Nunoi T, Takeda K, Matsumori A, Andoh M, Tsujinoue H, Nishimura K, Fukui H. Acute hemorrhagic colitis induced by the neuraminidase inhibitor oseltamivir. *Nippon Shokakibyo Gakkai Zasshi.* 2006 Nov;103(11):1270-3.

[37] Angelava NA, Angelava AV. Epidemiology, clinical picture, prevention and treatment of Avian influenza. *Georgian Med. News.* 2006 Feb;(131):69-76.

[38] Karatzios C, Gauvin F, Egerszegi EP, Tapiero B, Buteau C, Rivard GE, Ovetchkine P. Systemic capillary leak syndrome presenting as recurrent shock. *Pediatr. Crit. Care Med.* 2006 Jul;7(4):377-9.

[39] Grose C, Chokephaibulkit K. Avian influenza virus infection of children in Vietnam and Thailand. *Pediatr. Infect. Dis. J.* 2004;23:793-4.

[40] Chotpitayasunondh T, Lochindarat S, Srisan P. Cases of Influenza A (H5N1) - Thailand, 2004. *W. Epidemiol. Surveil. Rep.* 2004;5:100-103.

[41] Chotpitayasunondh T, Lochindarat S, Srisan P. Preliminary clinical description of influenza A (H5N1) in Thailand. W Epidemiol Surveil Rep 2004; 35: 89-92.

[42] Chokephaibulkit K, Uiprasertkul M, Puthavathana P, Chearskul P, Auewarakul P, Dowell SF, Vanprapar N. A child with avian influenza A (H5N1) infection. *Pediatr. Infect. Dis. J.* 2005;24:162-6.

[43] Centers for Disease Control and Prevention (CDC). Cases of influenza A (H5N1)-- Thailand, 2004. *MMWR Morb. Mortal. Wkly Rep.* 2004;53:100-3.

[44] Apisarnthanarak D. FIC Article Center, Atypical avian influenza (H5N1). Available at http//www.flu.org.cn

[45] Chan PK. Outbreak of avian influenza A(H5N1) virus infection in Hong Kong in 1997. *Clin. Infect. Dis.* 2002;34 Suppl 2:S58-64

[46] Brydak LB. Neurological complication of influenza infections. *Przegl. Epidemiol.* 2002;56 Suppl 1:16-30.

[47] Kamimura N, Matsuzaka T, Tsuji Y. Neurological outcome associated with influenza viral infection. *Nippon Rinsho.* 1997 Apr;55(4):880-5.

[48] Rybicka K, Brydak LB. Encephalopathy and encephalitis--influenza-associated neurological sequels. *Pol. Merkur. Lekarski.* 2005 Oct;19(112):501-5.

[49] Togashi T, Matsuzono Y, Narita M. Epidemiology of influenza-associated encephalitis-encephalopathy in Hokkaido, the northernmost island of Japan. *Pediatr. Int.* 2000 Apr;42(2):192-6.

[50] Rowe T, Cho DS, Bright RA, Zitzow LA, Katz JM. Neurological manifestations of avian influenza viruses in mammals. *Avian Dis.* 2003;47(3 Suppl):1122-6.

[51] Govorkova EA, Rehg JE, Krauss S, Yen HL, Guan Y, Peiris M, Nguyen TD, Hanh TH, Puthavathana P, Long HT, Buranathai C, Lim W, Webster RG, Hoffmann E. Lethality to ferrets of H5N1 influenza viruses isolated from humans and poultry in 2004. *J. Virol.* 2005 Feb;79(4):2191-8.

[52] Pappas DE, Owen Hendley J. Otitis media. A scholarly review of the evidence. *Minerva Pediatr.* 2003 Oct;55(5):407-14.

[53] Sugiura Y, Ohashi Y, Esaki Y, Furuya H, Ohno Y, Nakai Y. Influenza A virus-induced mucociliary dysfunction of tubotympanum. *Nippon Jibiinkoka Gakkai Kaiho.* 1991 Apr;94(4):506-15.

[54] Tong HH, Grants I, Liu X, DeMaria TF. Comparison of alteration of cell surface carbohydrates of the chinchilla tubotympanum and colonial opacity phenotype of Streptococcus pneumoniae during experimental pneumococcal otitis media with or without an antecedent influenza A virus infection. *Infect. Immun.* 2002 Aug;70(8):4292-301.

[55] Tong HH, Grants I, Liu X, DeMaria TF. Comparison of alteration of cell surface carbohydrates of the chinchilla tubotympanum and colonial opacity phenotype of Streptococcus pneumoniae during experimental pneumococcal otitis media with or without an antecedent influenza A virus infection. *Infect. Immun.* 2002 Aug;70(8):4292-301.

[56] Wiwanitkit V. Renal insufficiency on presentation of bird flu infection: is it correlated to outcome? *Clin. Exp. Nephrol.* 2006 Mar;10(1):87-8.

[57] Wiwanitkit V. Level of blood creatinine in the recent reported cases of bird flu infection in Thailand and Vietnam. *Nephrology* (Carlton). 2005 Aug;10(4):425.

[58] To KF, Chan PK, Chan KF, Lee WK, Lam WY, Wong KF, Tang NL, Tsang DN, Sung RY, Buckley TA, Tam JS, Cheng AF. Pathology of fatal human infection associated with avian influenza. A H5N1 virus. *J. Med. Virol.* 2001;63:242–6.

[59] Wiwanitkit V. Human bird flu infection: is there any relationship to hypertension? *Hypertension.* 2006 Jun;47(6):e28.

[60] Podolec P, Kopec G. Influenza vaccines for prevention of cardiovascular diseases. *Kardiol. Pol.* 2007 May;65(5):612-5.

[61] Antarasena C, Sirimujalin R, Prommuang P, Promkuntod N, Prommuang P, Blacksell SD. The indirect immunofluorescence assay using cardiac tissue from chickens, quails and ducks for identification of influenza A virus during an outbreak of highly pathogenic avian influenza virus (H5N1): a rapid and simple screening tool for limited resource settings. *Res. Vet. Sci.* 2007 Oct;83(2):279-81.

[62] Wiwanitkit V. Humans infected with bird flu: Is there evidence of cardiac disorder? *Can. J. Cardiol.* 2006 Jun;22(8):661.

[63] Erov NK. Diagnosis of infectious-allergic polyarthritis. *Revmatologiia* (Mosk). 1984 Jul-Sep;(3):60-2.

[64] Tsuruoka H, Xu H, Kuroda K, Hosaka Y. Viremia in influenza: detection by polymerase chain reaction. *Nippon Rinsho.* 1997 Oct;55(10):2714-8.

[65] Wiwanitkit V. Anemia in the recent reported cases of bird flu infection in Thailand and Vietnam. *J. Infect.* 2005 Oct;51(3):259.

[66] Wiwanitkit V. Platelet count in reported cases of bird flu infection in Thailand. *Platelets.* 2005 May-Jun;16(3-4):227.

[67] Wiwanitkit V. Hematologic Manifestations of Bird Flu, H5N1, *Infection. Infect Dis. Clin. Prac.* 2006 Jan; 14(1):9-11.

Chapter 6

Pathology of Bird Flu Infection

Genetic Mutation of Influenza Virus: A Possible Pathogenesis of New Bird Flu Infection [1 - 14]

Basically, an expression or phenotype is the final result of genotype. DNA is the starting point. DNA will signal via mRNA for protein synthesis in cytoplasm and further expression. The expression due to viral infection also follows this rule. After transfection or viral infection into the nucleus, infected cells undergo the described process to cause pathological expression. In a simple viral infection, known expression is well documented in medicine and proper treatment can be managed. However, problems will occur in cases of unknown expression due to viral mutation.

Simply, from DNA to expression, a signal pattern can be determined following mathematical principles. The possibility of error can be expected. In influenza, the mutation is considered an important factor that can lead to global pandemic. Basically there are two important types of mutations. The first is genetic or antigenic shift and the second is genetic or antigenic drift. Antigenic shift is a severe mutation process that can cause significant pathologic expression. This can lead to cross species infection. An example of antigenic shift occurs in shift mutation. Considering antigenic drift, mild changes can be seen. Sometimes it becomes silent a mutation. In the case of influenza, antigenic shift is common. Antigenic drift cannot bring the new subtype of influenza. Point mutation is a common cause of antigenic shift. Substitution, deletion or insertion can be identified in the case of antigenic shift. In influenza virus, RNA polymerase without proof reading actively contains errors at a rate of $1/10^4$ bases for each replication cycle. Mutated virus can be generated every day, but most of mutated viruses are nonsense and have no clinical implication.

A pandemic due to antigenic shift is expected in influenza in a case of combined strains of influenza virus infection in a single host. For example, a human infected with both human influenza and bird flu is at high risk for generation of a new genetic-shift virus. A reassortment of two influenza viral strains can be expected. Pandemic can be imagined in the event that the new combined influenza virus contains genes relating to infectivity and spreading properties for the new host, such as a new H5N1 virus combined with genes relating to human cell infectivity.

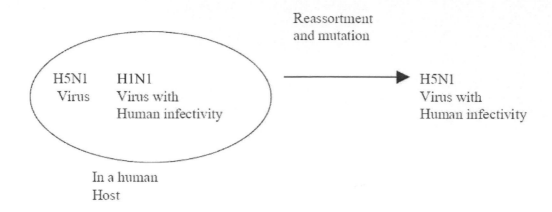

Figure 1. Diagram showing development of a new problematic H5N1 viral strain that can cause pandemic in human populations.

Pandemics due to reassortment and mutation have occurred in history. The well-known Asian flu (H2N2) in 1997 is a case study [19 – 22]. The H2N2 virus was the product of gene reassortment and mutation between human H1N1 virus and bird flu H2N2. The derived mutated H2N2 acquired NA, HA and PB, genes from H2N2 and five other segments from H1N1. Another example is Hong Kong flu (H3N2) in 1968 [23 – 32]. The mutated H3N2 was the result of combination between human H2N2 and bird flu (H3Nx). The derived H3N2 virus acquired PB1 and HA genes from bird flu, and other segments from humans. The mixing process of both generated a combined mutated virus that is expected to occur within swine. Swine (or pigs) are believed to be important mixing hosts for pandemic strains because pigs have cellular receptors for both HA from bird flu and human influenza viruses. It should be noted that only a simple point mutation in HA can significantly change the receptor birding specificity from alpha 2, 3-linked sugar to alpha 2, 6-linked sugar that is specific to humans. In addition, there are some reports indicating that PB2 mutation can also increase the ability of multiplication of virus in mammalian cells which can consequently increase the pathology. Wiwanitkit recently studied HA cleavage site mutation in bird flu virus in Thailand and proposed its relation to pathogenic degree and need for further surveillance [33]. According to the recent study by Viseshakul et al., molecular characterization of the avian H5N1 hemagglutinin (HA) gene was studied and the pattern "PQREKRRKKR" was proposed to be highly pathogenic [34]. Here, the author performed a similarity search for quoted pattern in the reported case of possible human-to-human transmission in Thailand (A/Thailand/ Kamphaengphet-Nontaburi/04(H5N1)) and the result showed that there is no matched quoted pattern. The mutation at the HA clevage site might not be a main factor contributing to the possible human-to-human transmission in Thailand.

As a conclusion, mutation of the virus is believed to be an important factor in causing a bird flu pandemic [35]. Presently, prediction of protein nanostructure and function is a great challenge in the proteomics and structural genomics era. To identify the point vulnerable to mutation is a new trend in expanding knowledge of disorders in the genomic and proteomic level of diseases [36 - 37]. Generally, disordered regions in proteins often contain short linear peptide motifs that are important for protein function. Identification of the peptide motifs in the amino acid sequence can give a good prediction for the weak linkages in a protein [36 - 37]. Here, the author performed a bioinformatics analysis to study the determine positions that trend to comply peptide motifs in the amino acid sequence of bird flu (H5N1) hemagglutinin. The database ExPASY [38] was used for searching for the amino acid sequence of H5N1 hemagglutinin. Then the derived sequences were used for further study of weak linkage. To identify the weak linkage in H5N1 hemagglutinin, a new bioinformatics tool named GlobPlot [39] was used. GlobPlot is a web service that allows the user to plot the tendency within the query protein for order/globularity and disorder [39]. It successfully identifies inter-domain segments containing linear motifs, and also apparently ordered regions that do not contain any recognized domain [39]. In this work, H5N1 hemagglutinin (A/Pheasant/Hong Kong/FY155/01 (H5N1)) was used for further study. For this H5N1 hemagglutinin, there were 68 positions identified in this study. The identified positions are presented in Figure 1. The positions 91-100, 128-142, 279-301, and 350-369 are identified as the position resistant to mutation.

In many infectious disease, the structural aberration is believed to be the main underlying pathogenesis. Some disorders are mentioned as a single substitution with other effects on the sequence frame; the others are mentioned as a frameshift. The mutations in H5N1 hemagglutinin are believed to be the possible starting point for further pandemics of bird flu. Here, the author used an algorithm to identify the positions in the amino acid sequences of H5N1 hemagglutinin that can be mutated. The author identified many positions. Some are known positions and others are newly discovered. Here, it can be shown that a simple diagnostic test for a single known mutation within H5N1 hemagglutinin cannot be the answer for successful controlling of bird flu infection. Also, it might imply the possibility for the occurrence of escape mutants that cannot be detected by the present standard PCR test. Based on this study, the weak linkages in the H5N1 hemagglutinin can be identified and can provide good information for predicting possible new mutations that can lead to a pandemic of H5N1 infection. In addition, the results of this study provide information for further research on the diagnosis of mutated bird flu and vaccine development.

slvksdqici gyhannsteq vdtimeknvt vthaqdilek thngklcdld gvkplilrdc svagwllgnp mcdefinvpe wsyivekasp ANDLCYPGDF ndyeelkhll srinhfckiq iipksswSNH EASSGVSSAC PYlgkssffr nvvwlikknn ayptikrsyn ntnqedllvl wgihhpndaa eqtklyqnpt tyisvgtstl nqrlvpkiat rskvngqsgr meffwtilkp ndainfesng nfiapeyayk ivkkgdsaim kseleygnCN TKCQTPMGAI NSSMPFHNIH Pltigecpky vksnrlvlat glrntpqrer rrkkrglfga iagfieggwQ GMVDGWYGYH HSNEQGSGYa adkestqkai dgvtnkvnsi idkmntqfea vgrefnnler rienlnkkme dgfldvwtyn aellvlmene rtldfhdsnv knlydkvrlq lrdnakelgn gcfefyhkcd necmesvkng tydypqylrk aglnreeisg vklesmgtyq ilsiystvas slalaimvag lslwmcsngs lqcrici

Figure 1. Identified positions (in capital) that comply peptide motifs in amino acid sequence of H5N1 hemagglutinin.

However, based on the principle of molecular biology, the mutation of nucleotide alone does not mean the alternation of expression, which implies the infectivity in this case. The mutation may be a silent one or can cause structural aberration of a specific encoded protein, which can lead to alteration of protein expression. Here, the author used a bioinformatics technique to predict the secondary and tertiary structures of the HA of H5N1 isolated in Thailand.

Table 1. Complete sequences of H5N1 of HA isolated in Thailand

Code	Description	Natural host
DQ334776	(A/chicken/Thailand/Nontaburi/CK-162/2005(H5N1))	Yes
DQ334778	(A/quail/Thailand/Nakhon Pathom/QA-161/2005(H5N1))	Yes
DQ334760	(A/chicken/Thailand/Kanchanaburi/CK-160/2005(H5N1))	Yes
AY972541	(A/tiger/Thailand/CU-T6/04(H5N1))	No
AY972539	(A/tiger/Thailand/CU-T4/04(H5N1))	No
AY646175	(A/leopard/Suphanburi/Thailand/Leo-1/04(H5N1))	No
AY972567	(A/tiger/Suphanburi/Thailand/Ti-1/04(H5N1))	No
AY555153	(A/Thailand/2(SP-33)/2004(H5N1))	No
DQ236085	(A/pigeon/Thailand/KU-03/04(H5N1))	Yes
DQ236077	(A/cat/Thailand/KU-02/04(H5N1))	No
DQ083585	(A/Mynas/Ranong/Thailand/CU-209/04(H5N1))	Yes
DQ083584	(A/sparrow/Phang-Nga/Thailand/CU-203/04(H5N1))	Yes
DQ083583	(A/pigeon/Samut Prakan/Thailand/CU-202/04(H5N1))	Yes
DQ083578	(A/chicken/Ratchaburi/Thailand/CU-68/04(H5N1))	Yes
DQ083573	(A/white peafowl/Bangkok/Thailand/CU-29/04(H5N1))	Yes
DQ083565	(A/chicken/Saraburi/Thailand/CU-17/04(H5N1))	Yes
DQ083564	(A/white peafowl/Bangkok/Thailand/CU-16/04(H5N1))	Yes
DQ083563	(A/crow/Bangkok/Thailand/CU-15/04(H5N1))	Yes
DQ083551	(A/chicken/Bangkok/Thailand/CU-3/04(H5N1))	Yes
DQ076201	(A/Ck/Thailand/73/2004(H5N1))	Yes

```
    --HHHEHHHHHHE-----EEEEE--------H-HHHHH---E--H-HHHHH------
------EE----HH------------------EHHH---------------HHHHHHH
HHHH------EEE-----------E--------------HHHHHHHH------EEEE---
-----HHHEEE--------HHHH-------EEEEE----------HHH----------
-EEEEEEH-------E----------HHHHHHE------HE-----------------
-------E----------------HHHHE---------HHHH-----EEHHE-EEH---
--EE---E------------------H-HH---H-----EHH----HHHHHHHHHHHHH
HHHHHH---HHH-HHEHHHHHHHHHHHHHH--------------HHHHHHHH---HH--
--HHHEE------HHHH-----------HH-HHHHHHH----E-E--HEEEEEEEEEHH
HHHHHHEHHH---EEEE-------EE—
```

Figure 2. Predicted secondary structures of H5N1 of HA isolated in Thailand (secondary structure prediction: H = helix, E = strand, - = no prediction).

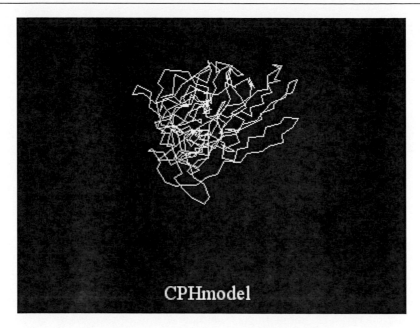

Figure 3. Predicted tertiary structures of H5N1 of HA isolated in Thailand.

Of interest, the structures of H5N1 derived from natural and non-natural hosts of the virus are the same. This implies that the mutation might not be the important factor leading to the cross species infection in Thailand, but rather the individual defect of the non-avian host might be the possible factor. Here, the author performed this study to compare the secondary and tertiary structures of the isolated HA from different sources in Thailand. The database PubMed was used for data mining of the nucleotide and amino acid sequences for HA of H5N1 isolated in Thailand. Only complete sequences were included for further study. The author performed protein secondary structure predictions of HA from its primary sequence using the NNPREDICT server [40]. Also, the author performed protein tertiary structure predictions of HA from its primary sequence using the CPHmodels 2.0 server [41].

The calculated secondary and tertiary structures were presented and compared. From searching the database PubMed, 20 complete sequences of H5N1 of HA isolated in Thailand were derived as shown in Table 1 (in February 2006). Using the NNPREDICT server, the calculation for the secondary structure of H5N1 of HA isolated in Thailand was performed. Using the CPHmodels 2.0 server, the calculation for the tertiary structure of H5N1 of HA isolated in Thailand was performed. The predicted structures of all 20 HA are the same. The predicted secondary and tertiary structures are shown in Figures 2 and 3, respectively.

Shinya and Kawaoka demonstrated that the epithelial cells in the upper respiratory tract of humans mainly possess sialic acid linked to galactose by alpha 2,6 linkages (SA alpha 2,6Gal), a molecule preferentially recognized by human viruses [42].

However, many cells in the respiratory bronchioles and alveoli possess SA alpha 2,3Gal, which is preferentially recognized by avian viruses [42]. These facts are consistent with the observation that H5N1 viruses can be directly transmitted from birds to humans and cause serious lower respiratory tract damage in humans [42]. The main action of H5N1 infection occurs after the complex formation between SA alpha Gal and H5N1 virus. It was found that SA-alpha-2, 3-Gal has strong multiple hydrophobic and hydrogen bond interactions in its trans conformation with H5N1 hemagglutinin, whereas the SA-alpha-2, 6-Gal only shows weak interactions in a different conformation (cis type) [43]. In this work, the author determines the change of binding energy between SA alpha Gal and H5N1 hemagglutinin due to the variation in rotatable angles.

As previously mentioned, binding between the SA alpha Gal and H5N1 hemagglutinin is the main reaction. The active side chain SA alpha Gal could be either 2,6Gal or 2,3Gal. The first Gal angle is fixed and the second Gal angle is variable. This is a calculation-based study. Basically, each chemical reaction poses it. Specific equired reaction energy is required. The primary assumption in this study is the required reaction energy for the reaction between each alpha Gal and H5N1 hemagglutinin is equal to 1 AkCal/mol when it occurs within a planar angle (interphase angle = 90 degrees). In this work, the theoretical simulation to find the difference in binding energy between 6Gal and 3Gal was performed. Calculation for the energy in each binding scenario was done based on physical theory of force. Based on basic geometry, the interGal angle (between the first fixed 2 Gal and the second Gal) was calculated. For the 3Gal, the interGal angle is equal to 60 degrees. For the 6Gal, the integral angle is equal to 240 degrees. These angle values were used for further simulating calculation for the binding energy. The summation of binding energy corresponding to the variation of second Gal angle is presented in Table 2. The derived binding energies difference is 1 A kcal/mol.

In nanomedicine, the consideration of the molecular interaction can give useful information to better understand the pathobiology of infection. The conformational analysis is a basic research technology that can be useful for explanation of the intermolecular , receptor - pathogen, interaction in an infection. Recently, Wiwanitkit reported the effect of conformational change of dihedral angle of TIBO on the effectiveness of HIV-RT [44]. There is some research to clarify the structure of SA alpha Gal and H5N1 hemagglutinin complex [43, 45 - 46]. However, there is no clarification on the conformation effect of SA alpha Gal variation on the receptor-pathogen interaction. In this research, the author tried to explain the energy difference corresponding to the conformational change within SA alpha Gal molecule. Here, the author found that the conformation variation within the SA alpha Gal molecule critically affects the binding energy. Decreased binding energy can be observed in 6 Gal. This implies the occurrence of reaction is easier in 6 Gal and further implies the higher infection. Based on the results in this study, it seems that 6 Gal is the more preferred receptor type for H5N1 transmission process.

Table 2. Summation of binding energy due to the variation of second Gal angle. Variation in second Gal Binding energy (kCal/mol)

Variation in second Gal	Binding energy (kCal/mol)
3 Gal	1.5 A
6 Gal	0.5 A

* The first 2 Gal is fixed

Indeed, conversion from SAalpha2,3Gal to SAalpha2,6Gal recognition is thought to be one of the changes that must occur before avian influenza viruses can replicate efficiently in humans and acquire the potential to cause a pandemic. This theory can be confirmed by the results from this study.

However, in addition to mutation, there is some evidencesthat bird flu can affect human without recruitment and mutation process. There were several instances of direct infection for H5N1, H9N2, H7N7, H7N3 and H10N7. The new query for these incidents is if there is a receptor mutation in those infected cases that brought high susceptibility to the direct infection.

Anatomical Pathology of Bird Flu

There is an interesting term that is used for describing the pathology in bird flu infection, pathotype. Pathotype is the term used to define the groups of avian influenza infection based on the pathological characteristics. There are two pathotypes of avian influenza infection, high pathogenic avian influenza and low pathogenic avian influenza. For high pathogenic avian influenza, there are many pathological appearances, both macroscopic and microscopic pathology, and the rate for fatality is high. On the other hand, for low pathogenic avian influenza, there are only a few pathological appearances, both macroscopic and microscopic pathology, and the rate for fatality is low. For the recent epidemic of H5N1, the high pathogenic avian influenza pathotype can be observed. The details of macroscopic and microscopic pathology for the H5N1 infection in the recent epidemic will be further discussed in this section.

A. Macroscopic Pathology

In avian influenza, the most frequently observed macroscopic lesions included: hemorrhages under the epicardium, in the proventricular and duodenal mucosa and pancreas; focal necrosis in the pancreas; myocardial degeneration; acute mucous enteritis; congestion of the spleen and lung, and the accumulation of sero-mucinous exudate in the body cavity [47]. Elbers et al. said that if peritonitis, or tracheitis, or edema of the neck and/or wattles or (petechial) haemorrhages in the proventriculus as observed at postmortem examination, especially if accompanied by an anamnesis describing acute and high mortality in a flock, this should consistently result in follow-up action to exclude highly pathogenic avian influenza in the differential diagnosis as cause of the disease problems by testing tissue samples with an avian influenza-specific laboratory test at the avian influenza reference laboratory [48].

For H5N1 infection in humans, To et al. studied 18 cases of human influenza A H5N1 infection identified in Hong Kong from May to December 1997 [49]. A full post-mortem showed reactive hemophagocytic syndrome as the most prominent feature [49]. Other findings included organizing diffuse alveolar damage with interstitial fibrosis, extensive hepatic central lobular necrosis, acute renal tubular necrosis and lymphoid depletion [49]. To et al. suggested that the pathogenesis of influenza A H5N1 infection might be different from that of the usual human subtypes H1-H3 [49]. Ng et al. said that H5N1 caused a more fulminant and necrotizing diffuse alveolar damage with patchy and interstitial paucicellular fibrosis compared to severe acute respiratory syndrome (SARS) [50]. In addition to lung lesion, edema and degeneration of myocytes in the heart and extensive acute tubular necrosis in the kidney can be observed.

To study the pathobiology, Nishimura et al. infected mice (ddY strain, 4 weeks old) intranasally with the H5N1 influenza viruses A/Hong Kong/156/97 (HK156) and A/Hong Kong/483/97 (HK483) isolated from humans [51]. According to this work, virus antigen could be detected by immunohistology in the heart and liver, albeit sporadically, but caused no degenerative change in these organs [51]. Of interest, the antigen was not detected in the thymus, spleen, pancreas, kidney or gastrointestinal tract but virus antigen was found frequently in adipose tissues attached to those organs and the adipose tissues showed severe degenerative change and the virus titers in the tissues were high and comparable to those in the lungs [50]. Nishimura et al. proposed that H5N1 influenza infection was pneumo-, neuro- and adipotropic, but not pantropic [51].

B. Microscopic Pathology

In birds, the microscopic pathology of avian flu can be well demonstrated in the neurological system. Microscopic lesions and detection of viral antigen can be confined to the central nervous system of the affected bird. In the cerebrum and to a minor extent in the brain stem a lymphohistiocytic meningoencephalitis with disseminated neuronal and glial cell necrosis, perivascular cuffing, glial nodules as well as focally extensive liquefactive necrosis can be observed [52]. In addition to the neurological system, the change can be well demonstrated in the respiratory system, microscopic lesions including moderate to severe serofibrinous pneumonia with severe pulmonary congestion can be observed [53]. For other systems, splenic changes including fibrin deposition and severe congestion, and severe congestion in kidneys can be seen [53].

For humans, apoptosis can be observed in alveolar epithelial cells, which is the major target cell type for the viral replication [54]. Uiprasertkul said that suggests that apoptosis may play a major role in the pathogenesis of influenza H5N1 virus in humans by destroying alveolar epithelial cells [54]. Histiocytic hyperplasia and hemophagocytic phenomena in lymphoid organs can also be seen [55].

C. Clinical Pathology of Bird Flu

In addition to anatomical pathology of bird flu, there are some interesting reports on the clinical pathology of flu. The details of important reports concerning clinical pathology of bird flu in the recent epidemic of H5N1 are hereby summarized in Table 3.

Table 3. The details of important reports concerning clinical pathology of bird flu in the recent epidemic of H5N1

Authors	Details
Wiwanitkit [56]	In this study, anemia, defined by hemoglobin level, in the recent reported cases of bird flu infection in Thailand and Vietnam was studied. It could be seen that anemia is common in bird flu infection.
Wiwanitkit [57]	In this study, renal insufficiency on presentation of bird flu infection, defined by the definition of blood chemistry test, was studied. It could be demonstrated that renal insufficiency on presentation of bird flu infection was related to the outcome of infection.
Wiwanitkit [58]	In this study, level of blood creatinine in the recent reported cases of bird flu infection in Thailand and Vietnam was studied. The hypercreatininemia could be observed in H5N1 infection.
Wiwanitkit [59]	In this study, the author studied the prothrombin time in reported cases of bird flu infection in Thailand and Vietnam. According to this work, prolonged prothrombin time was not common in bird flu infection.
Wiwanitkit [60]	In this study, the author studied the platelet count in reported cases of bird flu infection in Thailand and Vietnam. The author concluded that thrombocytopenia was an important hematological finding in reported cases of bird flu infection in Thailand.
Wiwanitkit [61]	In this study, the author studied the ratio of CD4+ to CD8+ T-Cells in the recent reported cases of bird flu infection in Asia. According to this work, similar finding on CD4+ and CD8+ to general influenza infection could be seen.
Wiwanitkit [62]	In this study, lymphocyte - neutrophil ratio on recent cases of bird flu infection in Thailand and Vietnam was studied. According to this work, considering the average and mean of reported lymphocyte – neutrophil ratios in bird flu cases, the trend of normal to increased ratio can be seen.

References

[1]   Meulemans G. Inter-species transmission of the influenza virus. *Bull. Mem. Acad. R. Med. Belg.* 1999;154(5-6):263-70

[2]   Kendal AP. Epidemiologic implications of changes in the influenza virus genome. *Am. J. Med.* 1987 Jun 19;82(6A):4-14.

[3]   Rott R. Influenza, a special form of zoonosis. *Berl Munch Tierarztl Wochenschr.* 1997 Jul-Aug;110(7-8):241-6.

[4]   Day T, Andre JB, Park A. The evolutionary emergence of pandemic influenza. *Proc. Biol. Sci.* 2006 Dec 7;273(1604):2945-53.

[5] Steensels M, Van Borm S, Van den Berg TP. Avian influenza: mini-review, European control measures and current situation in Asia. *Verh. K. Acad. Geneeskd. Belg.* 2006;68(2):103-20.

[6] Nishijima Y, Umeda M. Pandemic influenza measures in Japan--from the point of government. *Nippon Rinsho.* 2006 Oct;64(10):1781-8.

[7] Woo PC, Lau SK, Yuen KY. Infectious diseases emerging from Chinese wet-markets: zoonotic origins of severe respiratory viral infections. *Curr. Opin. Infect. Dis.* 2006 Oct;19(5):401-7.

[8] Chang SC, Cheng YY, Shih SR. Avian influenza virus: the threat of a pandemic. *Chang Gung Med. J.* 2006 Mar-Apr;29(2):130-4.

[9] Angelava NA, Angelava AV. Epidemiology, clinical picture, prevention and treatment of Avian influenza. *Georgian Med. News.* 2006 Feb;(131):69-76.

[10] Webster RG, Hulse DJ. Microbial adaptation and change: avian influenza. *Rev. Sci. Tech.* 2004 Aug;23(2):453-65.

[11] Okabe N. The possibility and preparedness for pandemic of new influenza. *Nippon Rinsho.* 2003 Nov;61(11):1904-8.

[12] Shigeta S. Recent progress in anti-influenza chemotherapy. *Drugs R. D.* 1999 Sep;2(3):153-64.

[13] Cox NJ, Subbarao K. Global epidemiology of influenza: past and present. *Annu. Rev. Med.* 2000;51:407-21.

[14] Stephenson I, Zambon M. The epidemiology of influenza. *Occup. Med.* (Lond). 2002 Aug;52(5):241-7.

[15] Subbarao K, Luke C. H5N1 viruses and vaccines. PLoS Pathog. 2007 Mar;3(3):e40.

[16] Allen PJ. Avian influenza pandemic: not if, but when. *Pediatr. Nurs.* 2006 Jan-Feb;32(1):76-81.

[17] Wong SS, Yuen KY. Avian influenza virus infections in humans. *Chest.* 2006 Jan;129(1):156-68.

[18] Liu JP. Avian influenza--a pandemic waiting to happen? *J. Microbiol. Immunol. Infect.* 2006 Feb;39(1):4-10.

[19] Levine R. A cure for the Asian flu. *Biosecur Bioterror.* 2006;4(3):228-30.

[20] Kilbourne ED. Influenza pandemics: past, present and future. *J. Formos. Med. Assoc.* 2006 Jan;105(1):1-6.

[21] Schafer JR, Kawaoka Y, Bean WJ, Suss J, Senne D, Webster RG. Origin of the pandemic 1957 H2 influenza A virus and the persistence of its possible progenitors in the avian reservoir. *Virology.* 1993 Jun;194(2):781-8.

[22] Nerome K, Yoshioka Y, Torres CA, Oya A, Bachmann P, Ottis K, Webster RG. Persistence of Q strain of H2N2 influenza virus in avian species: antigenic, biological and genetic analysis of avian and human H2N2 viruses. *Arch. Virol.* 1984;81(3-4):239-50.

[23] Cockburn WC, Delon PJ, Ferreira W. Origin and progress of the 1968-69 Hong Kong influenza epidemic. *Bull. World Health Organ.* 1969;41(3):345-8.

[24] Buescher EL, Smith TJ, Zachary IH. Experience with Hong Kong influenza in tropical areas. *Bull. World Health Organ.* 1969;41(3):387-91.

[25] Chang WK. National influenza experience in Hong Kong, 1968. *Bull. World Health Organ.* 1969;41(3):349-51.

[26] White PC Jr. A2-Hong Kong-68. *Va Med Mon* (1918). 1968 Oct;95(10):595-6.

[27] Hrabar A, Ugrcic I. A-2 Hong Kong influenza epidemic in Croatia in 1969-70. *Lijec. Vjesn.* 1972 Mar;94(3):125-31.

[28] Kundin WD. Hong Kong influenza. Serological, immunochemical and epidemiologic studies. *Taiwan Yi Xue Hui Za Zhi.* 1969 Nov 28;68(11):568-9.

[29] Davis LE, Caldwell GG, Lynch RE, Bailey RE, Chin TD. Hong Kong influenza: the epidemiologic features of a high school family study analyzed and compared with a similar study during the 1957 Asian influenza epidemic. *Am. J. Epidemiol.* 1970 Oct;92(4):240-7.

[30] Influenza: the Hong Kong virus. *WHO Chron.* 1968 Dec;22(12):528-9.

[31] Vastag B. Hong Kong flu still poses pandemic threat. *JAMA.* 2002 Nov 20;288(19):2391-5.

[32] Hong Kong influenza: the coming winter. *Med. J. Aust.* 1970 Feb 21;1(8):393-4.

[33] Wiwanitkit V. HA cleavage site mutation in bird flu virus in Thailand: relation to pathogenic degree and further surveillance. *Am. J. Infect. Control.* 2006 Sep;34(7):468.

[34] Viseshakul N, Thanawongnuwech R, Amonsin A, Suradhat S, Payungporn S, Keawchareon J, Oraveerakul K, Wongyanin P, Plitkul S, Theamboonlers A, Poovorawan Y. The genome sequence analysis of H5N1 avian influenza A virus isolated from the outbreak among poultry populations in Thailand. *Virology.* 2004;328:169-76.

[35] Trampuz A, Prabhu RM, Smith TF, Baddour LM. Avian influenza: a new pandemic threat? *Mayo Clin. Proc.* 2004;79:523-30

[36] Lee C, Wang Q. Bioinformatics analysis of alternative splicing. *Brief Bioinform.* 2005;6:23-33

[37] Levin JM, Penland RC, Stamps AT, Cho CR. Using in silico biology to facilitate drug development. *Novartis Found Symp.* 2002;247:222-38

[38] 4. Gasteiger E, Gattiker A, Hoogland C, Ivanyi I, Appel RD, Bairoch A. ExPASy: The proteomics server for in-depth protein knowledge and analysis. *Nucleic Acids Res.* 2003;31:3784-8.

[39] Linding R, Russell RB, Neduva V, Gibson TJ. GlobPlot: Exploring protein sequences for globularity and disorder. *Nucleic Acids Res.* 2003 ;31:3701-8

[40] Kneller DG, Cohen FE, Langridge R. Improvements in Protein Secondary Structure Prediction by an Enhanced Neural Network. *J. Mol. Biol.* 1990; 214: 171-182.

[41] Lund O, Nielsen M, Lundegaard C, Worning P. CPHmodels 2.0: X3M a Computer Program to Extract 3D Models," Abstract at the CASP5 conferenceA102, 2002.

[42] Shinya K, Kawaoka Y. Influenza virus receptors in the human airway. *Uirusu.* 2006;56:85-9.

[43] Li M, Wang B. Computational studies of H5N1 hemagglutinin binding with SA-alpha-2, 3-Gal and SA-alpha-2, 6-Gal. *Biochem. Biophys. Res Commun.* 2006 Sep 1;347(3):662-8.

[44] Wiwanitkit V. Analysis of binding energy activity of TIBO and HIV-RT based on simple consideration for conformational change. *African J. Biotech.* 2007; 6: 188-189.

[45] Yamada S, Suzuki Y, Suzuki T, Le MQ, Nidom CA, Sakai-Tagawa Y, Muramoto Y, Ito M, Kiso M, Horimoto T, Shinya K, Sawada T, Kiso M, Usui T, Murata T, Lin Y, Hay A, Haire LF, Stevens DJ, Russell RJ, Gamblin SJ, Skehel JJ, Kawaoka Y. Haemagglutinin mutations responsible for the binding of H5N1 influenza A viruses to human-type receptors. *Nature*. 2006 ;444:378-82.

[46] Stevens J, Blixt O, Tumpey TM, Taubenberger JK, Paulson JC, Wilson IA. Structure and receptor specificity of the hemagglutinin from an H5N1 influenza virus. *Science*. 2006 Apr21;312(5772):404-10.

[47] Pálmai N, Erdélyi K, Bálint A, Márton L, Dán A, Deim Z, Ursu K, Löndt BZ, Brown IH, Glávits R. Pathobiology of highly pathogenic avian influenza virus (H5N1) infection in mute swans (Cygnus olor). *Avian Pathol*. 2007 Jun;36(3):245-9.

[48] Elbers AR, Kamps B, Koch G. Performance of gross lesions at postmortem for the detection of outbreaks during the avian influenza A virus (H7N7) epidemic in The Netherlands in 2003. *Avian Pathol*. 2004 Aug;33(4):418-22.

[49] To KF, Chan PK, Chan KF, Lee WK, Lam WY, Wong KF, Tang NL, Tsang DN, Sung RY, Buckley TA, Tam JS, Cheng AF. Pathology of fatal human infection associated with avian influenza A H5N1 virus. *J. Med. Virol*. 2001 Mar;63(3):242-6.

[50] Ng WF, To KF, Lam WW, Ng TK, Lee KC. The comparative pathology of severe acute respiratory syndrome and avian influenza A subtype H5N1--a review. *Hum. Pathol*. 2006 Apr;37(4):381-90.

[51] Nishimura H, Itamura S, Iwasaki T, Kurata T, Tashiro M. Characterization of human influenza A (H5N1) virus infection in mice: neuro-, pneumo- and adipotropic infection. *J. Gen. Virol*. 2000 Oct;81(Pt 10):2503-10.

[52] Klopfleisch R, Werner O, Mundt E, Harder T, Teifke JP. Neurotropism of highly pathogenic avian influenza virus A/chicken/Indonesia/2003 (H5N1) in experimentally infected pigeons (Columbia livia f. domestica). *Vet. Pathol*. 2006 Jul;43(4):463-70.

[53] Ficken MD, Guy JS, Gonder E. An outbreak of influenza (H1N1) in turkey breeder hens. *Avian Dis*. 1989 Apr-Jun;33(2):370-4.

[54] Uiprasertkul M. Apoptosis and Pathogenesis of Avian Influenza A (H5N1) Virus in Humans. *Emerg. Infect Dis*. 2007 May;13(5):708-12.

[55] Zhang W, Wen LY, Lu M, Xiong Y, Qian KJ, Deng AH, Guo LS, Xiao ZK, Zhao XS, Duan SM, Xie ZG, Gao ZF, Li M, Shao HQ, Wang GG, Liu DW, Gao ZC. Clinical characteristic analysis of the first human case infected by influenza A (H5N1) in Jiangxi Province. *Zhonghua Jie He He Hu Xi Za Zhi*. 2006 May;29(5):300-6.

[56] Wiwanitkit V. Anemia in the recent reported cases of bird flu infection in Thailand and Vietnam. *J. Infect*. 2005 Oct;51(3):259.

[57] Wiwanitkit V. Renal insufficiency on presentation of bird flu infection: is it correlated to outcome? *Clin. Exp. Nephrol*. 2006 Mar;10(1):87-8.

[58] Wiwanitkit V. Level of blood creatinine in the recent reported cases of bird flu infection in Thailand and Vietnam. *Nephrology* (Carlton). 2005 Aug;10(4):425

[59] Wiwanitkit V. Prolonged prothrombin time is not common in bird flu infection: a summary from Thailand. *J. Thromb. Haemost*. 2005 Sep;3(9):2127-8.

[60] Wiwanitkit V. Platelet count in reported cases of bird flu infection in Thailand. *Platelets*. 2005 May-Jun;16(3-4):227.

[61] Wiwanitkit V. Ratio of CD4+ to CD8+ T-Cells in the recent reported cases of bird flu infection in Asia. *Iran J. Immunol.* 2007 Mar;4(1):58-60.

[62] Wiwanitkit V. Lymphocyte - neutrophil ratio on recent cases of bird flu infection in Thailand and Vietnam. *Internet J. Infect. Dis.* 2005;4(2): 1.

Chapter 7

Laboratory Investigation for Bird Flu Infection

Specimen Collection and Processing for Bird Flu Suspected Cases [1 – 6]

Given the limitations for routine surveillance, including variations in the interval between illness onset and specimen capture, the quality of the swab, delays in transport [5 - 6], good specimen collection and processing for bird flu suspected cases is needed. Upon initial suspicion of A/H5N1, similar procedures are recommended. An epidemiologic investigation is necessary to specify whether the patient stayed in a country where A/H5N1 virus was circulating. Clinical samples needed for a specific diagnosis are: nasopharyngeal, throat-swab or fecal samples, cerebrospinal fluid and blood. However, the specimen from respiratory tract is widely used since bird flu is a respirator infection [7].

A. Specimen Collection

In cases of an epidemic of animal deaths with bird flu infection as the suspected cause, a forensic diagnosis is needed. The basic principles for collection of victims' bodies are:

1) Since bird flu infection is considered an emerging infectious disease, a report to the local Center of Disease Control (CDC) is needed.
2) The specimen collection and destruction of the dead animals' bodies for further necropsy and laboratory study should be under the control of CDC specialists. The techniques for specimen collection are listed in Table 1.
3) Collected specimens in sealed plastic bags should be opened in a specific hood in a specific laboratory.
4) The personnel who take action at specimen reception must use all protective devices as previously described.

Table 1. Technique for specimen collection

Recommended	Not recommended
Gown, mask, goggle and gloves are needed.	No protective equipment
Healthy adult collector is needed.	Childhood or geriatric collector
Dead bodies of animals must be collected in sealed water protected plastic bags and kept in ice.	Use of non-sealed plastic bag
Prompt delivery of collected sample to the laboratory is recommended.	Delayed delivery
Disinfectant must be applied to the site after specimen collection.	No disinfectant
Body cleaning after specimen collection is recommended for all collections.	No body cleaning after specimen collection

5) In case the whole body cannot be collected, important parts such as the pancreas, lung and spleen can be autopsied and collected then transported to the laboratory. The amount of specimen should be 5 grams per organ.

In cases of a living suspected animal, different specimen collection techniques can be applied. The recommended techniques are swabbing techniques.

Swabbing is recommended. Collector should swab the mucosal secretions from the nostil, trachea cloacal slit or cloaca using a specific polyester swab. The collected swab must be kept in 1-2 cc of viral transport media, be labeled and promptly transferred in ice to the laboratory.

For suspected human case, the nostril and tracheal swabbing can be applied. In addition, tracheal lavage and bronchoalveolar lavage can be used for specimen collection. The collector must use the principle of infection control for respiratory infection protocol and universal precautions during specimen collection process. In addition, chemoprophylaxis by oseltaminir must be used.

B. Transportation of Specimen

The specimen should be promptly delivered to the laboratory. The sealed plastic bag containing the specimen should be kept in a ice and placed in closed sunlight-protected container. The period of delivery should be less than 24 hours. In cases that the sample must be refrigerated, it can be kept in a refrigerator for 48 hours. In case of prolonged keeping, deep freezing at -70°C is recommended. In a deep freezing condition, the collected sample can be kept for 1 month.

C. Analytical Process

The analytical process must be performed in a specific virology laboratory. It should be noted that the laboratory for analysis of animal samples must not be in the same place as the laboratory for analysis of human samples. The standard laboratory quality control is needed.

Table 2. Swabbing techniques

Animals	Recommended techniques
Mammal	Nostril and tracheal swabbing
Avian	Cloacal slit or cloaca swabbing

In addition, protocol for high risk emerging infectious disease must be used. The details of present diagnostic method will be presented in the next heading.

Diagnostic Methods for Bird Flu Virus

There are many diagnostic methods for bird flu virus. The details of important diagnostic methods will be presented and discussed.

1. Viral Culture Method [8 - 10]

Bird flu virus can be cultured in an egg or specific cell culture, Madin – Darby Canine Kidney (MDCK), Rhesus monkey kidney or epithelial cell LLC-MK2. The technique for culture starts from centrifugation of sample collection tube. Separated supernatant will be used for further laboratory process. In case the collected sample is tissue, homogenate preparation must be performed before centrifugation. The details of insulation and culture are different due to type of culture.

1.1. Egg Culture

The culture process starts from inoculation of 0.15-0.3 CC of prepared sample into 9 to 11 days-hatched embryonated egg. The inoculation must be directly to the allantion sac. At least three eggs should be inoculated per one prepared sample. The inoculated eggs must be kept at 37°C for 72 hours. Apply lamp light to test the viability of the embryos within the eggs two times per day. At 72 hours, collection of all fluids aspirated from allantion sacs of the three eggs will be done. The collected fluid will be firstly tested for hemagglutinin. If positive, exclusion for Newcastle disease virus must be done. After ruling out of Newcastle disease virus, positive fluid will be further tested by RT-PCR or real time PCR. The problem of egg culture is the complicated culture technique. Poor inoculation technique can lead to a false negative. Another limitation of this technique is the long turnaround time (at least 3 days). In addition, the bio-safety level 3 laboratory is needed for this type of culture.

According to this culture system, the level of lactic dehydrogenase activity is an indicator of the growth of influenza virus in the embryonate egg [11].

1.2. MDCK Cell Culture [12 – 13]

The 48 hours MDCK cell culture is required. The prepared sample will be applied into the well plate containing cell culture. Continuous observation for 72 hours must be performed. In a positive cause the cytopathogenic effects of swelling and demarcation of the cell culture can be observed. Meguro et al. said that the cell line proved more sensitive than either eggs or rhesus monkey cells for currently circulating influenza A and B strains [14]. Meguro et al. said that influenza viruses caused a distinct cytopathology within 5 days of inoculation if trypsin-ethylenediamine-tetraacetic acid was incorporated into the medium [14]. Hornickova showed that the influenza B strain had a greater cytotoxic effect on MDCK cells than influenza A [15]. Hornickova proposed that a higher infection dose of influenza A virus accelerated the onset of apoptosis; conversely, a higher infection dose of influenza B virus delayed the onset of apoptosis [15]. Sufficient hemagglutinin was produced on the initial tissue culture passage to allow direct identification of isolates by hemagglutinin inhibition tests. Persistent influenza virus infection in a MDCK cell culture was confirmed [16]. This technique is widely used for human sample. The centrifugation assay is a rapid and specific method for detection of influenza A and B viruses in clinical specimens, and it can serve as a valuable and cost-efficient adjunct to conventional culture methods [17]. Positive cell must be further tested by PCR technique. However, Frank et al. said that MDCK was less useful for parainfluenza viruses [18]. Brands et al. concluded that this cell line and the cell culture system were suitable for biological production from the characterization of the continuous cell line MDCK as well as drug safety studies [19].

1.3. LLC-MK2 Culture [20]

LLC-MK2 is another widely used cell line for respiratory virus culture. It comes from a monkey kidney. The effect of oleic acid [21] and isomeric cis-octadecenoic acids [22] on the growth of LLC-MK2 was proposed for a long time. This is confirmed as a good viral cell culture [23]. Frank reported that LLC-MK2 was much superior to MDCK for parainfluenza viruses [24].

2. Immunological Method

There are several immunological methods for detection of bird flu virus. The common methods will be hereby discussed.

2.1. Immunofluorescence Assay (IFA) [25]

This technique requires a specific fluorescence microscope. The positive cell will be coded by a fluorescence-stained antibody. Nucleus and cytoplasmic illumination under fluorescence microscope indicates a positive finding. Ray and Minnich studied efficiency of immunofluorescence for rapid detection of common respiratory viruses [26]. According to this research, the sensitivity of FA for detection of parainfluenza virus type 1, parainfluenza virus type 3, influenza A virus, and adenoviruses ranged from 28 to 63%, but specificities for these viruses were uniformly 98 to 100% [26]. Minnich and Ray performed a study to compare direct immunofluorescent staining of clinical specimens for respiratory virus antigens with conventional isolation techniques [27]. According to this work, of 292 patients who were culture positive for these viruses, 259 were diagnosed by detection of the viral antigen in clinical specimens by direct immunofluorescence [27]. No specimens that subsequently yielded a different respiratory virus by culture were positive by the direct immunofluorescence method [27]. Minnich and Ray concluded that the study of selected antisera based on clinical history of the patient reduced the cost of rapid viral diagnosis [27]. A new rapid direct immunofluorescence assay (DFA) respiratory screen reagent for detection of seven common respiratory viruses (respiratory syncytial virus [RSV], influenza A and B viruses, parainfluenza virus types 1 to 3, and adenovirus) was recently launched [28]. Landry and Ferguson said that the availability of a rapid DFA screening reagent for detection of multiple common respiratory viruses within 1 to 2 h of sample collection should be of great benefit in terms of patient management and infection control [28].

2.2. Hemagglutination and Hemagglutination Inhibition Test [29 - 30]

Basically, hemagglutinin protein can agglutinate red blood cells. Hemagglutination inhibition test is based on the reaction of antisera for prevention of agglutination. Specific antisera can be applied for subtype classification of influenza virus. A favorable sensitivity and specific for diagnosis of influenza by hemagglutination and hemagglutination inhibition test was reported [31]. Korneeva et al. said that the sensitivity and specificity of the proposed test was found to be equal to those of the serological and immunofluorescent methods but to be more advantageous than the latter in the simplicity of its performance and demonstrative results [32]. A receptor destroying enzyme (RDE) preparation is an additional technique to increase the efficacy of hemagglutination and hemagglutination inhibition test for influenza diagnosis [33]. In addition, Halon et al. also reported that the sensitivity of the hemagglutination-inhibition test for influenza was significantly increased by the addition of species-specific anti-immunoglobulin G serum [34].

2.3. Serology Test

Similar to general influenza infection serological test can be used for diagnosis of human infection. Pour serum can be used. The general serological techniques for bird flu virus detection include virus neutralization test and enzyme-linked immunosorbant assay (ELISA). Neutralization test for influenza has a long history [35 – 36]. Neutralization antibodies are important defenses in influenza infection [37 - 39]. Jayasekara et al. said that natural IgM and the early components of the classical pathway of complement worked in concert to neutralize influenza virus and that this interaction might have a significant impact on the course of influenza viral pneumonia [40]. Knossow et al. reported that neutralization occurred at an average of one antibody bound per four hemagglutinins, a ratio sufficient to prevent the simultaneous receptor binding of hemagglutinins that is necessary to attach virus to cells. There are several methods for detection of neutralization antibodies [41]. In 1999, Bachmann et al. described novel in vitro assays to determine influenza virus titers and virus neutralizing antibody levels [42]. This assay made it possible to distinguish between IgM and IgG antibody titers and was about 5-10 fold more sensitive than a classical hemagglutination inhibition assay using fresh chicken blood [42].

ELISA is a widely used technique for diagnosis of influenza [43]. In 1979, an enzyme-linked immunosorbent assay (ELISA) using horseradish peroxidase was described by Lambre and Kasturi for the detection and quantitation of anti-influenza virus antibodies [44]. According to this work, ELISA's sensitivity, closed to that of radioimmunoassay permits detection of small amounts of antibodies in pulmonary secretions and supernatants from in vitro spleen cell cultures [44]. A rapid and easy purification method was developed to obtain avian influenza antigen for use in immunochemical assays was described by Abraham et al. in 1984. Rabbit anti-turkey globulins were made specific for turkey globulins, using affinity chromatography, conjugated to horseradish peroxidase and used in enzyme-linked immunosorbent assay [45]. This purified antigen eliminated the false-positives from ELISA for avian influenza detection [45]. In 1985, Snyder et al. developed a new ELISA for detecting antibody to type A avian influenza virus. Under field conditions, this ELISA was able to detect serum avian influenza antibody in flocks from which highly pathogenic avian influenza was isolated [46]. A double-antibody sandwich ELISA (DAS-ELISA) was developed for detection of avian influenza virus antigen in 1993 by Kodihalli et al. [47]. Kodihalli et al. reported that percentage agreement between indirect DAS-ELISA and virus isolation in AIV-positive samples was found to be 76.1% and, in avian influenza virus-negative samples, it was found to be 82.1% [47]. These results indicate that the DAS-ELISA might be a viable alternative to virus isolation because of its rapidity, compared with virus isolation [47]. In the same year, Kodihalli et al. also developed an antigen-capture ELISA for rapid diagnosis of avian influenza virus in commercial turkey flocks [48]. In 1998, Shafer et al. developed a competitive enzyme-linked immunosorbent assay (CELISA) using a baculovirus vector, Autographa californica nuclear polyhedrosis virus, expressing the nucleoprotein (NP) gene of A/Ann Arbor/6/60 influenza virus [49]. Shafer et al. proposed that the CELISA was a rapid, economical, sensitive, and specific serodiagnostic method for screening large numbers of avian sera for antibodies to avian influenza virus [49]. In 1998, a competitive enzyme-linked immunosorbent assay (C-ELISA) employing a baculovirus-expressed recombinant nucleoprotein and a monoclonal antibody was developed for the detection of antibodies to type A influenza virus nucleoprotein by Zhou et al. [50]. Zhou et al. proposed that C-ELISA had the potential to replace the agar gel immunodiffusion test for screening sera from avian species, including ratites, for detection of antibodies to type A influenza virus [50]. In 2003, a one-tube reverse transcriptase/polymerase chain reaction coupled with an enzyme-linked immunosorbent assay (RT-PCR-ELISA) was developed for the rapid detection of avian influenza virus (AIV) in clinical specimens by Dybkaer et al. [51]. Dykbaer et al. said that the diagnostic sensitivity and specificity of the RT-PCR-ELISA was 91% and 97%, respectively, using virus isolation in specific pathogen-free eggs as the gold reference standard [51].

2.4. Antigen Detection

Antigen detection is an alternative in diagnosis of influenza [52]. Passive hemagglutination test is an example of antigen detection method for diagnosis of influenza [53]. Immunofluorescence is another described technique [54]. Recently, Chen et al.

developed a rapid and simple latex agglutination test (LAT) for the detection of avian influenza virus (AIV) subtype H5N1 in chicken allantoic fluids, tracheal swabs, and tissues [55]. According to this method, monoclonal antibodies against the hemagglutinin glycoprotein of H5N1 are covalently coupled onto the surface of carboxylated latex bead using a water-soluble carbodiimide to obtain sensitized latex particles (SLP) [55]. When the LAT was compared with other detection methods, the agreement with the viral isolation, H5 antigen immunochromatographic test, and H5 real-time RT-PCR test was 93.97, 95.18, and 87.95%, respectively [55].

3. Molecular Biology Based Method

Molecular biology based methods are widely used for diagnosis of bird flu at present. The polymerase chain reaction (PCR) is the main principle for most molecular biology based methods. PCR is rapid and has high sensitivity. Before PCR procedure, the sample had to be harvested from allantoic fluid or cell culture. The sample will be extracted for RNA and reverse transcription is the performed. Basically PCR contains the following steps. Firstly, house-keeping gene is identified. This step is to confirm that the specimen is from the affected host. This is necessary to confirm that there is no false negative and the sample is extracted from the affected host. Secondly, a matrix (M) gene will be detected. The M gene is specific for all subtypes of influenza A virus. The positive result means that there is influenza A virus in the sample and further laboratory analysis is needed. Thirdly, hemaglutinin gene (H gene) is identified. This is for classification of subtypes to H1 to H6. Finally, a neuraminidase gene (N gene) is identified. This is for further classification of subtypes N1 to N9. With this four step protocol, the subtype of influenza virus can be determined. Several different methods, including traditional RT-PCR, real-time RT-PCR, and nucleic acid sequence-based amplification among others, have been described for the diagnosis of avian influenza in poultry with many different variations of primers, probes, enzymes. In 2002, Poddar reported influenza virus types and subtypes detection by single step single tube multiplex reverse transcription-PCR (RT-PCR) and agarose gel electrophoresis [56]. Poddar noted that the sensitivity of detection was about 0.01 TCID(50) for both influenza type A and B when amplification was for typing alone while the sensitivities for types and subtypes specific bands were 0.01-0.1 TCID (50) in the tested volume in multiplex subtyping or multiplex typing and subtyping simultaneously [56]. A 5'-nuclease real-time reverse transcriptase-polymerase chain reaction assay was developed by Whiley and Sloots for the detection of influenza type A and was validated using a range of influenza A subtypes, including avian strains in 2005 [57].

For bird flu, the specific M, H5 and N1 gene expressed as 680 bp, 350 bp and 160 bp lines on electrophoresis. However, there is a newly developed method for direct detection of virus from collected sample without cell culture. This can help fasten the turnaround time of diagnosis. In 2006, Payungporn et al. developed a multiplex real-time RT-PCR for rapid detection of H5N1 influenza A virus [58]. The selected primer set was used in single-step RT-PCR for simultaneous detection in multiplex format of the 276-, 189-, and 131-bp fragments, corresponding to sequences specific for M, H5 and N1 [59]. The amplified DNA fragments were clearly separated by agarose gel electrophoresis [59]. The results showed that the multiplex real-time RT-PCR assays could be applied to detect virus suspensions of H5N1 influenza A virus from a wide host range and demonstrated the sensitivity of the assay amounted to approximately 10^2-10^3copies/ml [58]. In conclusion, the highlights of this particular method lie in its rapidity, specificity and sensitivity thus rendering it feasible and effective for large-scale screening at times of H5N1 influenza A virus outbreaks [58]. In 2006, Wei et al. developed another single-step multiplex RT-PCR for H5N1 diagnosis [60]. Wei et al. suggested that the method was rapid and specific and, therefore, could be valuable in the rapid detection of H5N1 influenza viruses in clinics [60]. In 2006, Ng et al. also developed another one-step RT- PCR assay to detect the H5N1 avian influenza A virus [61]. Detection was 100% from allantoic fluid in H5N1 positive samples, suggesting it to be a reliable sampling source for accurate detection [61].

In addition, the pathotype of H5N1 can also be determined by PCR technique. The high and low pathogenic strains can be discrete at cleavage site of hemagglutinin. In 2006, a diagnostic kit for detection of avian influenza virus by real-time polymerase chain reaction was developed by Bisiuk et al. [62]. The diagnostic kit is universal and adopted for ABI PRISM SDS (Applied Biosystems), RotorGene (Corbett Research) and iQCycler (BioRad) PCR machines [62]. The high pathogenic strain contains arginine and lysine residues and this makes the trypsin easier cut this cleavage site. Real time PCR can be applied for discrimination purpose. In 2007, Hoffmann et al. developed a new real-time RT-PCR assay which enabled sensitive and specific detection and cleavage site analysis of high pathogenic H5N1 of the Qinghai lineage [63]. In 2007, Chen et al. also described another sensitive and specific real-time RT-PCR method for the detection of influenza A subtype H5 and for monitoring virus loads [64]. The melting temperature can also be used as a cut off for pathotype classification. The H5 gene of high pathogenic strain melts at 77.43 degree Celcius while that of low pathogenic strain melts at 79.57 degree Celcius (cut-off value equals 78.50 degree Celcius).

4. Rapid Test for Bird Flu

Early diagnosis is a concept in secondary prevention. Early diagnosis can help hasten treatment of an affected case and infection control can be promptly set [65]. There are many rapid tests for bird flu at present. Molecular diagnostic tests are commonly used to diagnose avian influenza virus because they are sensitive and can be performed rapidly, with high throughput, and at a moderate cost [66]. Molecular diagnostic tests recently have proven themselves to be invaluable in controlling disease outbreaks around the world [66]. However, those PCR-based methods cannot be used as a rapid test in the field. A point-of-care testing for influenza might be a better solution for filed survey. Rapid influenza tests are increasingly used in surveillance systems and for clinical care. However, the performance and utility of rapid influenza tests under field conditions has not been fully evaluated. Poehling et al. performed interesting research to determine whether a point-of-care rapid influenza test impacts the diagnostic evaluation and treatment of children with acute respiratory illnesses [67]. They proposed that point-of-care rapid influenza tests were sensitive and specific and were associated with less diagnostic testing in the emergency department [67]. Simmerman et al. said that rapid influenza tests were useful to describe the seasonality of influenza, estimate the cost of illness, increase the sensitivity of surveillance, conduct outbreak responses, and guide evaluation of suspected avian influenza virus infections [68].

References

[1]   Thongcharoen P. Bird's flu. Siriraj Hosp Gaz. 1998; 50(6): 631-638.
[2]   Platinavin L. Avian influenza (bird flu) *W. Epidemiol. Surveil. Rep.* 2004 Jan; 35(4): 49-52.
[3]   Sangka A. Avian flu or bird flu viruses. *J. Med. Technol. Phys. Ther.* 2004 Jan-Dec; 16 (1-3): 14-21.
[4]   Srithamma S, Sangkitporn S, Thawatsupha P, Auwanit W, Chitakanpitch M, Waicharoen S, Kitphati R. Coordinating system for testing and laboratory surveillance for bird flu, Department of Medical Sciences, Ministry of Public Health. *Bull. Dept. Med. Sci.* 2005 Apr-Jun; 47 (2): 124-138.
[5]   Fleming DM. Influenza diagnosis and treatment: a view from clinical practice. *Philos. Trans. R. Soc. Lond B. Biol. Sci.* 2001 Dec 29;356(1416):1933-43.
[6]   L'vov DK, Slepushkin AN, Iamnikova SS, Burtseva EI. Influenza remains an unpredictable infection. *Vopr. Virusol.* 1998 May-Jun;43(3):141-4.
[7]   Goffard A, Lazrek M, Schanen C, Lobert PE, Bocket L, Dewilde A, Hober D. Emergent viruses: SARS-associate coronavirus and H5N1 influenza virus. *Ann. Biol. Clin.* (Paris). 2006 May-Jun;64(3):195-208.
[8]   Haque A, Lucas B, Hober D. Influenza A/H5N1 virus outbreaks and prepardness to avert flu pandemic. *Ann. Biol. Clin.* (Paris). 2007 Mar-Apr;65(2):125-33.
[9]   Booy R, Brown LE, Grohmann GS, Macintyre CR. Pandemic vaccines: promises and pitfalls. *Med. J. Aust.* 2006 Nov 20;185(10 Suppl):S62-5.
[10]   Zambon M. Cell culture for surveillance on influenza. *Dev .Biol. Stand.* 1999;98:65-71.
[11]   Kelly R, Greiff D. The level of lactic dehydrogenase activity as an indicator of the grwoth of influenza virus in the embryonate egg. *J. Exp. Med.* 1961 Jan 1;113:125-9.
[12]   Nakamura K, Nishizawa S. Isolation of influenza virus by use of MDCK cell suspension (author's transl). *Kansenshogaku Zasshi.* 1979 Dec;53(12):698-703.
[13]   Nakamura K, Nishizawa S. Method of suspension culture for MDCK cells and isolation of influenza virus in MDCK suspension cultured cells (author's transl). *Kansenshogaku Zasshi.* 1980 Jun;54(6):306-12.
[14]   Meguro H, Bryant JD, Torrence AE, Wright PF. Canine kidney cell line for isolation of respiratory viruses. *J. Clin. Microbiol.* 1979 Feb;9(2):175-9.
[15]   Hornickova Z. Different progress of MDCK cell death after infection by two different influenza virus isolates. *Cell Biochem. Funct.* 1997 Jun;15(2):87-93.b
[16]   Medvedeva MN, Aron RA, Golubev DB. Persistent influenza virus infection in a MDCK cell culture. *Vopr. Virusol.* 1984 Sep-Oct;29(5):536-9.

[17] Mills RD, Cain KJ, Woods GL. Detection of influenza virus by centrifugal inoculation of MDCK cells and staining with monoclonal antibodies. *J. Clin. Microbiol.* 1989 Nov;27(11):2505-8.

[18] Frank AL, Couch RB, Griffis CA, Baxter BD. Comparison of different tissue cultures for isolation and quantitation of influenza and parainfluenza viruses. *J. Clin. Microbiol.* 1979 Jul;10(1):32-6.

[19] Brands R, Visser J, Medema J, Palache AM, van Scharrenburg GJ. Influvac: a safe Madin Darby Canine Kidney (MDCK) cell culture-based influenza vaccine. *Dev. Biol. Stand.* 1999;98:93-100.

[20] Hull RN, Cherry WR, Tritch OJ. Growth characteristics of monkey kidney cell strains LLC-MK1, LLC-MK2, and LLC-MK2(NCTC-3196) and their utility in virus research. *J. Exp. Med.* 1962 May 1;115:903-18.

[21] Jenkin HM, Anderson LE. The effect of oleic acid on the growth of monkey kidney cells (LLC-MK2). *Exp. Cell Res.* 1970 Jan;59(1):6-10.

[22] Jenkin HM, Anderson LE, Holman RT, Ismail IA, Gunstone FD. The effect of isomeric cis-octadecenoic acids on the growth of monkey kidney cells (LLC-MK2). *Exp. Cell. Res.* 1970 Jan;59(1):1-5.

[23] Cook RA, Counter FT, McColley JK. Characterization of a long-term suspension culture of the LLC-MK2 monkey kidney cell line. *In Vitro.* 1974 Mar-Apr;9(5):323-30.

[24] Frank AL. Selected laboratory aspects of influenza surveillance. *Yale J. Biol. Med.* 1982 May-Aug;55(3-4):201-5.

[25] Liu C. Immunofluorescent technic: application in the study and diagnosis of infectious diseases. *Clin. Pediatr.* (Phila). 1963 Sep;2:490-7.

[26] Ray CG, Minnich LL. Efficiency of immunofluorescence for rapid detection of common respiratory viruses. *J. Clin .Microbiol.* 1987 Feb;25(2):355-7.

[27] Minnich L, Ray CG. Comparison of direct immunofluorescent staining of clinical specimens for respiratory virus antigens with conventional isolation techniques. *J. Clin. Microbiol.* 1980 Sep;12(3):391-4.

[28] Landry ML, Ferguson D. SimulFluor respiratory screen for rapid detection of multiple respiratory viruses in clinical specimens by immunofluorescence staining. *J. Clin. Microbiol.* 2000 Feb;38(2):708-11.

[29] Solomon JM, Gibbs MB, Bowdler AJ. Methods in quantitative hemagglutination II. *Vox. Sang.* 1965 Mar-Apr;10:133-48.

[30] Potter CW, Oxford JS. Determinants of immunity to influenza infection in man. *Br. Med. Bull.* 1979 Jan;35(1):69-75.

[31] Beskrovnaia LA, Doborova IN, Korneeva EP, Baranov EN. Sensitivity and specificity of influenza diagnostic preparations for the indirect hemagglutination reaction. *Voen. Med. Zh.* 1980 Jan;(1):39-41.

[32] Korneeva EP, Shvartsman IaS, Gorenskaia RL, Shefer LF, Potapenko LB. Use of the indirect hemagglutination reaction for the express diagnosis of influenza outbreaks]. *Vopr. Virusol.* 1977 Sep-Oct;(5):628-32.

[33] Jordan WS Jr, Oseasohn RO. The use of RDE to improve the sensitivity of the hemagglutination-inhibition test for the serologic diagnosis of influenza. *J. Immunol.* 1954 Mar;72(3):229-35.

[34] Hahon N, Booth JA, Eckert HL. Anti-immunoglobulin G hemagglutination-inhibition test for influenza. *Infect. Immun.* 1971 Oct;4(4):508-10.

[35] Boyd MR. Neutralisation test for influenza virus using roller drums. *Ir. J. Med. Sci.* 1962 Jan;433:44-5.

[36] Sprossig M. Attempt of a neutralization test in a dysembryonated egg with influenza viruses. *Zentralbl Bakteriol* [Orig]. 1955 Nov;164(1-5):188-91.

[37] Gerhard W. The role of the antibody response in influenza virus infection. *Curr. Top. Microbiol. Immunol.* 2001;260:171-90.

[38] Dimmock NJ. Mechanisms of neutralization of animal viruses. *J. Gen. Virol.* 1984 Jun;65 (Pt 6):1015-22.

[39] Shvartsman YS, Zykov MP. Secretory anti-influenza immunity. *Adv. Immunol.* 1976;22:291-330.

[40] Jayasekera JP, Moseman EA, Carroll MC. Natural antibody and complement mediate neutralization of influenza virus in the absence of prior immunity. *J. Virol.* 2007 Apr;81(7):3487-94.

[41] Knossow M, Gaudier M, Douglas A, Barrere B, Bizebard T, Barbey C, Gigant B, Skehel JJ. Mechanism of neutralization of influenza virus infectivity by antibodies. *Virology.* 2002 Oct 25;302(2):294-8.

[42] Bachmann MF, Ecabert B, Kopf M. Influenza virus: a novel method to assess viral and neutralizing antibody titers in vitro. *J. Immunol. Methods.* 1999 May 27;225(1-2):105-11.

[43] Flewett TH. Rapid diagnosis of virus diseases. *Br. Med. Bull.* 1985 Oct;41(4):315-21.

[44] Lambre C, Kasturi KN. A microplate immunoenzyme assay for anti-influenza antibodies. *J. Immunol. Methods.* 1979;26(1):61-7.

[45] Abraham A, Sivanandan V, Newman JA, Maheswaran SK. Rapid purification of avian influenza virus for use in enzyme-linked immunosorbent assay. *Am. J. Vet. Res.* 1984 May;45(5):959-62.

[46] Snyder DB, Marquardt WW, Yancey FS, Savage PK. An enzyme-linked immunosorbent assay for the detection of antibody against avian influenza virus. *Avian Dis.* 1985 Jan-Mar;29(1):136-44.

[47] Kodihalli S, Sivanandan V, Nagaraja KV, Goyal SM, Halvorson DA. Antigen-capture enzyme immunoassay for detection of avian influenza virus in turkeys. *Am. J. Vet. Res.* 1993 Sep;54(9):1385-90.

[48] Kodihalli S, Sivanandan V, Halvorson DA, Nagaraja KV, Kumar MC. Antigen-capture ELISA for rapid diagnosis of avian influenza virus in commercial turkey flocks. *J. Vet. Diagn. Invest.* 1993 Jul;5(3):438-40.

[49] Shafer AL, Katz JB, Eernisse KA. Development and validation of a competitive enzyme-linked immunosorbent assay for detection of type A influenza antibodies in avian sera. *Avian Dis.* 1998 Jan-Mar;42(1):28-34.

[50] Zhou EM, Chan M, Heckert RA, Riva J, Cantin MF. Evaluation of a competitive ELISA for detection of antibodies against avian influenza virus nucleoprotein. *Avian Dis.* 1998 Jul-Sep;42(3):517-22.

[51] Dybkaer K, Munch M, Handberg KJ, Jorgensen PH. RT-PCR-ELISA as a tool for diagnosis of low-pathogenicity avian influenza. *Avian Dis.* 2003;47(3 Suppl):1075-8.

[52] Dwyer DE, Smith DW, Catton MG, Barr IG. Laboratory diagnosis of human seasonal and pandemic influenza virus infection. *Med. J. Aust.* 2006 Nov 20;185(10 Suppl):S48-53.

[53] Gorbunova AS, Sokovykh LI, Isachenko VA. Detection of viral and host antigens contained in an allantoic culture of influenza virus by means of the passive hemagglutination test. *Vopr. Virusol.* 1966 May-Jun;11(3):318-22.

[54] Lyarskaya TY, Ketiladze ES, Zhilina NN, Orlova NN. Detection of viral antigen by autoradiography and immunofluorescence in epithelial cells of the respiratory tract in natural and experimental influenza infection. *Acta Virol.* 1966 Nov;10(6):521-7.

[55] Chen J, Jin M, Yu Z, Dan H, Zhang A, Song Y, Chen H. A latex agglutination test for the rapid detection of avian influenza virus subtype H5N1 and its clinical application. *J. Vet. Diagn. Invest.* 2007 Mar;19(2):155-60.

[56] Poddar SK. Influenza virus types and subtypes detection by single step single tube multiplex reverse transcription-polymerase chain reaction (RT-PCR) and agarose gel electrophoresis. *J. Virol. Methods.* 2002 Jan;99(1-2):63-70.

[57] Whiley DM, Sloots TP. A 5'-nuclease real-time reverse transcriptase-polymerase chain reaction assay for the detection of a broad range of influenza A subtypes, including H5N1. *Diagn. Microbiol. Infect. Dis.* 2005 Dec;53(4):335-7.

[58] Payungporn S, Chutinimitkul S, Chaisingh A, Damrongwantanapokin S, Buranathai C, Amonsin A, Theamboonlers A, Poovorawan Y. Single step multiplex real-time RT-PCR for H5N1 influenza A virus detection. *J. Virol. Methods.* 2006 Feb;131(2):143-7.

[59] Payungporn S, Phakdeewirot P, Chutinimitkul S, Theamboonlers A, Keawcharoen J, Oraveerakul K, Amonsin A, Poovorawan Y. Single-step multiplex reverse transcription-polymerase chain reaction (RT-PCR) for influenza A virus subtype H5N1 detection. *Viral Immunol.* 2004;17(4):588-93.

[60] Wei HL, Bai GR, Mweene AS, Zhou YC, Cong YL, Pu J, Wang S, Kida H, Liu JH. Rapid detection of avian influenza virus a and subtype H5N1 by single step multiplex reverse transcription-polymerase chain reaction. *Virus Genes.* 2006 Jun;32(3):261-7.

[61] Ng LF, Barr I, Nguyen T, Noor SM, Tan RS, Agathe LV, Gupta S, Khalil H, To TL, Hassan SS, Ren EC. Specific detection of H5N1 avian influenza A virus in field specimens by a one-step RT-PCR assay. *BMC Infect. Dis.* 2006 Mar 2;6:40.

[62] Bisiuk IIu, Mel'nichuk SD, Oblap RV, Spiridonov VG, Martynenko DL, Mel'nichuk MD, Lisovenko VT. Development of diagnostic kit "Ptakh-Grip PLR" for detection of highly pathogenic strain of avian influenza virus H5N1 by polymerase chain reaction. *Mikrobiol. Z.* 2006 Jul-Aug;68(4):70-8.

[63] Hoffmann B, Harder T, Starick E, Depner K, Werner O, Beer M. Rapid and highly sensitive pathotyping of avian influenza A H5N1 virus by using real-time reverse transcription-PCR. *J. Clin. Microbiol.* 2007 Feb;45(2):600-3.

[64] Chen W, He B, Li C, Zhang X, Wu W, Yin X, Fan B, Fan X, Wang J. Real-time RT-PCR for H5N1 avian influenza A virus detection. *J. Med. Microbiol.* 2007 May;56(Pt 5):603-7.

[65] Dwyer DE, McPhie KA, Ratnamohan VM, Pitman CN. Challenges for the laboratory before and during an influenza pandemic. *N. S. W. Public Health. Bull.* 2006 Sep-Oct;17(9-10):142-5.

[66] Suarez DL, Das A, Ellis E. Review of rapid molecular diagnostic tools for avian influenza virus. *Avian Dis.* 2007 Mar;51(1 Suppl):201-8.

[67] Poehling KA, Zhu Y, Tang YW, Edwards K. Accuracy and impact of a point-of-care rapid influenza test in young children with respiratory illnesses. *Arch. Pediatr. Adolesc. Med.* 2006 Jul;160(7):713-8.

[68] Simmerman JM, Chittaganpitch M, Erdman D, Sawatwong P, Uyeki TM, Dowell SF. Field performance and new uses of rapid influenza testing in Thailand. *Int. J. Infect. Dis.* 2007 Mar;11(2):166-71.

Chapter 8

Aspect in Veterinarian Medicine for Bird Flu Infection

Outbreak of Avian Flu in Birds

It is recorded that there have been numerous outbreaks of avian flu in birds in the past. Since avian flu is a specific infection for birds, infection in birds can easily occur and outbreaks can be respected. The summary of documented outbreaks of avian flu in birds from 1950 to 2000 is summarized in Table 1.

Table 1. Outbreaks of bird flu from 1950 to 2000 [1 - 26]

Year	Country	Strain
1959	Scotland, UK	H5N1
1961	South Africa	H5N3
1963	UK	H7N3
1966	Canada	H5N3
1975	Australia	H7N7
1979	UK	H7N7
1983-1984	USA	H5N2
1983	Ireland	H5N8
1985	Australia	H7Nx
1991	UK	H7N3
1992	Australia	H7N3
1994	Australia	H5N2
1994-1995	Mexico	H5N1
1995	Pakistan	H7N3
1996	Hong Kong	H5N1
1997	Australia	H7N4
1997	Italy	H5N2
1999-2000	Italy	H7N1

It should be noted that most of the outbreaks from 1950 to 2000 occurred in Europe and the highly pathogenic strain of bird flu virus is the main cause. One of the possible explanations is that the viral isolation technique was not fully available in the past in Asia and there might have been other undetectable outbreaks of avian flu in birds in Asian during the mentioned period.

Principle for Destroying Dead Infected Animals

Since dead H5N1 infected animals can be the source of disease dissemination, good management of the dead animals is necessary. After complete specimen collection for necropsy and laboratory diagnosis, all corpses must be correctly destroyed. The recommended protocol for destroying dead infected animals is

1. The one who takes responsible for destroying the dead infected animal has to follow respiratory precautions and infection control principles [27 - 35]. The practitioners for this process must be well trained and should get bird flu chemoprophylaxis [36 - 41]. The practitioner has to wear gloves, gown, mask, cap and goggles [42].
2. The corpses should be incinerated in a specific heating apparatus or buried. The burial site should be prepared at the epidemic site [43]. Dig 2-5 meter deep burial sites and drop all corpses, feces, animal foods, eggs and all other nearby feeding apparatus and materials into the burial site. Cover the buried things with anti-infective agents, such as chlorine solution, properly. Close the burial site and protect the site with wooden or zinc plate to prevent opening by any scavengers.
3. Apply disinfectant around the burial site. Continuously wash and spray of disinfectant twice a day for a continuous three days
4. Destroy gloves, gown, mask, cap and goggles after use at burial site. Spray all other clothing with disinfectant. Change into new clothing before leaving the burial site.
5. All digging apparatus has to be cleaned and disinfected. All apparatus must not be moved out.

Table 2. "Don't" of destroying of dead infected animals

Don't
Destroying death infected animal with no protective apparatus
Throwing dead animals into the canal or river.
Abandoning the corpses at the epidemic site
Destroying without notification to local center of disease control or without specimen collection for necropsy for a laboratory diagnosis
Digging burial site near water reservoir
Selling dead animals or their eggs to the outside markets
Destroying done by low-educated personnel.
Leaving feces or animal parts without burying
Wearing gloves, gown, mask, cap and goggles out of the burial site.
Wearing same clothing out of the burial site after complete destruction process.

*As a conclusion, universal precautions should be strictly used [44 - 52].

Stability of H5N1 Virus in Chicken Product

It is confirmed that H5N1 is a respiratory virus [53 – 54]. The main mode of transmission is respiration. Closed contact with birds is the common history of human H5N1 infected cases. In infected birds, the virus can be detected in respiratory and gastrointestinal tracts but not in flesh. However, the main suspicion at present is if the virus can contaminate chicken meat. The transmission by ingestion has never been confirmed but widely discussed. The case of tiger H5N1 infection in Thailand [55 - 57] brings attention to the possible oral route of transmission of bird flu. Basically chicken products can be produced in several farming systems (in-house farming, medium farming and large farming). The H5N1 influenza virus in chickens has become a concern at present because there are some avian carriers without any symptoms in cases of an epidemic of H5N1 virus. If the farm is in-house farming or a small farm and lacks good protocol to detect a silent H5N1 infection, the silent infected chicken carrier can be killed by the farm owner and those killed chicken can be sold as chicken products to the community. However, in large farming with a well controlled system, the risk is scientifically decreased.

In addition to chicken flesh, the egg is another important product. Luckily, an H5N1 chicken usually decreases egg production. However, the possibility still exists. Nevertheless, the virus can contaminate the egg shell. These situations are also reported in many infectious diseases [58 - 61]. The contact with H5N1 containing feces from an infected chicken can be the cause of contamination of the egg shell. In this case, it can be a problematic source of H5N1 spreading. However, several environmental factors including temperature, sunlight and alkaline pH can help destroy the contaminated virus in the egg shell [62].

An important protocol in many chicken farms before distribution of eggs to the market is egg washing and sanitizing. This procedure can help decrease contamination in the egg shell. Previously, three methods of disinfection were commonly used in poultry houses: fumigation with formaldehyde, pulverization of an iodophore and synthetic phenols [63]. Egg washing is better than the previously widely used formalin fumigation [64 - 67]. The principle in egg washing is washing with water having a higher temperature than the eggs. The washed eggs should be abruptly dried. There is a present automatic system for egg washing. This automated system contains three chambers.

The first chamber is for washing with warm 43 degree Celsius water with anti-infective solution and detergent. The contaminated feces will be removed by water at this chamber. The second chamber is for rinsing with disinfectant such as quaternary ammonium and chlorine solution. The last chamber is for drying by heat wind or ultraviolet light. Connect washing, can help decrease germs on the egg shell and prolong shelf life of the egg. However, incorrect washing can increase contamination.

Table 3. Causes of the increase of contamination due to incorrect egg washing

Causes	Details
1. Prolonged Washing	Prolonged washing increases of possibility of contact with external microbes and prolongs the period of contact that can lead to increased chance of the microbial penetration into the egg shell.
2. Too much washing	Too much washing will decrease natural surfactant at egg shell and this can lead to an increased chance of the microbial penetration into the egg shell.
3. Too little washing	Too little washing leaves behind contaminated germs. If these eggs with contaminated germs were distributed into the market, it can be the main sources of germs spreading.

The recommended procedure for correct egg washing is listed below:

1. Wash all eggs. It is time consuming and not cost effective to select specific eggs with dirty appearance to wash. In addition, eggs with clean appeared might have unseen contamination.
2. Abruptly wash eggs after being laid down because it is easy to wash and decrease the opportunity of contact between external microbes and egg shells.
3. Use water with a higher temperature than the egg for washing. The recommended temperature of water is 10 degree Celsius more than the egg. This recommendation is to prevent negative pressure in the egg that can suck contamination inside egg.
4. Use sanitizer and detergent in addition to water. This process should be repeated two times.
5. Check for the expiration date and appearance of sanitizer and detergent before use.
6. Frequently change the water during washing. In addition, the water should be confirmed for low iron content because iron increases risk of germ growing in the eggs.
7. Abruptly dry washed eggs then pack eggs into the cartons. Delayed drying increases risk of microbes growing and increases evaporation that decreases quality of eggs.

As previously mentioned, germs can penetrate the egg shell into the egg. There are many related factors contributing to penetration. These factors will be further discussed.

1. Structure of egg shell

The egg shell has its main function in protection. The avian eggshell is a complex, extracellularly assembled structure which contains both mineralized and non-mineralized regions. The outer shell consists of cuticle while the inner shell consists of a small membrane. Although the egg shell is solid it is fragile and contains numerous microspores. After being laid down, egg shell is still soft. It takes a few moments for cuticle to set up and to impose its protection function. Inside the egg, albumin and yolk can be found. Tan et al. said that the diameter of the fibers of the inner layer of the egg membrane ranged from .08 to .64 microns, whereas those of the outer layer of the same membrane ranged from .05 to 1.11 microns [68].

Tan et al. noted that fibers in the shell membrane ranged from .11 to 4.14 microns diameter [68]. Carrino et al. suggested that the dermatan sulfate proteoglycans might be important in modulating crystal morphology in the hen eggshell and correlated with mineralization-modulating biomolecules from other calcified tissue, which were generally anionic [69]. Wiwanitkit recently performed a theoretical study to verify if avian bird flu virus can pass through the eggshell [70]. Because most viruses are approximately spherical, the virus is modeled as a sphere moving through the pore [70 – 71]. Its motion is influenced by convection in the carrier fluid, diffusion, and short-range interactions with the pore walls [70, 72]. Interactions that trap the virus against the pore wall are the primary barriers to transmission [70, 72]. This concept can be used for predicting the transmission of avian flu virus via eggshell. The author analyzed the feasibility of avian flu virus passing through the eggshell based on a consideration at the nanostructure level. The basic concept is that if the size of the virus is larger than the pore size of the eggshell, the virus cannot pass through the pores [70, 72]. Wiwanitkit searched for the sizes of the virus and the pores of eggshell in the literature [70]. The eggshell pore size is about 200 to 600 nm in diameter [70, 73] and the avian flu virus is about 100 nm [70, 73]. Based on the particle size as a single factor, the author hereby proposes that transmission of the studied viruses through the eggshell is feasible. Indeed, the passing of plague virus, a virus with similar size to the avian flu virus, has been confirmed for years [70, 74]. Therefore, there is no doubt that the avian flu virus can pass through the eggshell. Li et al. noted that although the source of these recently isolated Hong Kong 97-like H5N1 viruses was undetermined, their detection in the egg shell of duck and goose suggested that this particular genotype of H5N1 virus might have re-emerged in nature or might have been circulating continuously [75].

2. Negative pressure

After being laid, the egg still has a higher temperature than the environment. However, for a while, the temperature decrease and this brings negative pressure. The negative pressure can suck nearby particles inside and this can be the period when germs could be sucked into the egg. This is an important fact and has already been mentioned in the egg washing process.

3. Moisture

Moisture eases the transmission of germs from external site to internal side of egg [76]. Moisture can be the result of sweating, which can be due to rapid change of egg's temperature and environmental temperature. Sweating is common in the case of a hatching machine. Sweating accompanied with negative pressure increase opportunity of germ contamination through egg shell. Smith et al. reported that increasing excreta moisture gave a linear increase in the (log-transformed) numbers of microorganisms that contaminated ostensibly clean egg shells [77].

4. Microbe or germ

If there is no microbe or germ, the problem will not occur. Since an egg can easily to be contact the chicken's feces, the contact with germs cannot be avoided. Sanitization at a chicken farm is necessary. Proper egg washing should be applied.

Good Management of Chicken Flesh

Good management of chicken flesh focuses on every stage starting from farming by farm owners to eating by the general public. During farming, sanitation can be good for the health of the chicken. The risk can start from the infection with H5N1 virus by a farmed chicken. If these infected chickens become silent carriers, they put at risk the workers who slaughter the chickens because they can come in contact with the virus during the chicken killing process. It is suggested that killing chickens should be performed in a well-controlled, clean place. The killer should be educated and wear good protective apparatus. In the Muslim culture, the chicken killer must be well trained and wash themselves before killing the chicken. This can decrease the risk of viral contact. As previously mentioned, the internal organs of the chicken are a high risk for viral contamination. Gastrointestinal and respiratory visceral organs can be sources of an H5N1 virus. These organs should not be ingested in the situation of H5N1 epidemic. The chicken killer who comes in contact with these visceral organs must wash their hands and change clothes after the killing. There are some reported human H5N1 cases among the local population who act as chicken killers in home farming. This is considered as a high-risk contact [78 - 79].

Regarding ingestion of chicken flesh, there is no report of H5N1 transmission by this mode. The well-done chicken flesh is safe, however, rare or medium-cooked chicken flesh is high risk. The recommendation for cooking chicken flesh before ingestion is cooking the flesh until its internal temperature reaches at least 70 degree Celsius. Make sure that heat can enter into the deep center of the chicken flesh. For an egg, it should be heated at 60 degree Celsius for at least 3.5 minutes. A summary on safe ingestion of chicken product is listed in Table 4.

Of interest, there was a recent report on contamination of bird flu virus in chicken flesh. Tumpey et al. noted that the DK/Anyang/AVL-1/01 virus was unique among the H5N1 isolates in that infectious virus and viral antigen could also be detected in muscle and brain tissue of ducks [80]. Tumpey et al. said that the isolation of a highly pathogenic H5N1 influenza virus from poultry indicated that such viruses were still circulating in China and may present a risk for transmission of the virus to humans [80]. Tumpey et al. also noted that the presence of an H5N1 influenza virus in ducks bearing a hemagglutinin gene that was highly similar to those of the pathogenic 1997 human/poultry H5N1 viruses raised the possibility of reintroduction of highly pathogenic avian influenza to chickens and humans [81]. Lu et al. compared the Dk/Anyang virus with highly pathogenic H5N1 viruses isolated from humans in 1997 in terms of antigenicity and pathogenicity for mammals [82]. Lu et al. reported that compared with highly pathogenic human H5N1 viruses, Dk/Anyang virus is substantially less pathogenic for mammalian species [82]. Lu et al. also reported that A/Dkmt virus cross-reacted poorly with ferret antisera raised against human H5N1 viruses, but prior infection with A/Dkmt virus protected mice from death after secondary infection with human H5N1 virus [83].

Table 4. A summary on safe ingestion of chicken products

Suggestions
Thoroughly cook chicken flesh and eggs before ingestion.
Refrigerating or freezing cannot destroy H5N1 virus.
Washing can decrease but not destroy H5N1 virus.
Do not ingest raw or medium cooked chicken products.
Don't share the kitchenware for preparing raw and cooked foods.
Egg from farm passing egg washing needs no additional wash.

References

[1]   Wood JM, Webster RG, Nettles VF. Host range of A/Chicken/Pennsylvania/83 (H5N2) influenza virus. *Avian Dis.* 1985 Jan-Mar;29(1):198-207.

[2]   Kawaoka Y, Naeve CW, Webster RG. Is virulence of H5N2 influenza viruses in chickens associated with loss of carbohydrate from the hemagglutinin? *Virology.* 1984 Dec;139(2):303-16.

[3]   Nettles VF, Wood JM, Webster RG. Wildlife surveillance associated with an outbreak of lethal H5N2 avian influenza in domestic poultry. *Avian Dis.* 1985 Jul-Sep;29(3):733-41.

[4]   Cappucci DT Jr, Johnson DC, Brugh M, Smith TM, Jackson CF, Pearson JE, Senne DA. Isolation of avian influenza virus (subtype H5N2) from chicken eggs during a natural outbreak.*Avian Dis.* 1985 Oct-Dec;29(4):1195-200.

[5]   Wood JM, Kawaoka Y, Newberry LA, Bordwell E, Webster RG. Standardization of inactivated   H5N2   influenza   vaccine   and   efficacy   against   lethal A/Chicken/Pennsylvania/ 1370/83 infection. Avian Dis. 1985 Jul-Sep;29(3):867-72.

[6]   Webster RG, Kawaoka Y, Bean WJ. Vaccination as a strategy to reduce the emergence of amantadine- and rimantadine-resistant strains of A/Chick/Pennsylvania/83 (H5N2) influenza virus. *J. Antimicrob. Chemother.* 1986 Oct;18 Suppl B:157-64.

[7]   Donatelli I, Campitelli L, Di Trani L, Puzelli S, Selli L, Fioretti A, Alexander DJ, Tollis M, Krauss S, Webster RG. Characterization of H5N2 influenza viruses from Italian poultry. *J. Gen. Virol.* 2001 Mar;82(Pt 3):623-30.

[8]   De Marco MA, Foni E, Campitelli L, Delogu M, Raffini E, Chiapponi C, Barigazzi G, Cordioli P, Di Trani L, Donatelli I. Influenza virus circulation in wild aquatic birds in Italy during H5N2 and H7N1 poultry epidemic periods (1998 to 2000). *Avian Pathol.* 2005 Dec;34(6):480-5.

[9]   Capua I, Marangon S, dalla Pozza M, Terregino C, Cattoli G. Avian influenza in Italy 1997-2001. *Avian Dis.* 2003;47(3 Suppl):839-43.

[10]   Mutinelli F, Capua I, Terregino C, Cattoli G. Clinical, gross, and microscopic findings in different avian species naturally infected during the H7N1 low- and high-pathogenicity avian influenza epidemics in Italy during 1999 and 2000. *Avian Dis.* 2003;47(3 Suppl):844-8.

[11] Mannelli A, Ferre N, Marangon S. Analysis of the 1999-2000 highly pathogenic avian influenza (H7N1) epidemic in the main poultry-production area in northern Italy. *Prev. Vet. Med.* 2006 Mar 16;73(4):273-85.

[12] Mulatti P, Kitron U, Mannelli A, Ferre N, Marangona S. Spatial analysis of the 1999-2000 highly pathogenic avian influenza (H7N1) epidemic in northern Italy. *Avian Dis.* 2007 Mar;51(1 Suppl):421-4.

[13] Di Trani L, Bedini B, Cordioli P, Muscillo M, Vignolo E, Moreno A, Tollis M. Molecular characterization of low pathogenicity H7N3 avian influenza viruses isolated in Italy. *Avian Dis.* 2004 Apr-Jun;48(2):376-83.

[14] Lu H, Dunn PA, Wallner-Pendleton EA, Henzler DJ, Kradel DC, Liu J, Shaw DP, Miller P. Investigation of H7N2 avian influenza outbreaks in two broiler breeder flocks in Pennsylvania, 2001-02. *Avian Dis.* 2004 Jan-Mar;48(1):26-33.

[15] Dunn PA, Wallner-Pendleton EA, Lu H, Shaw DP, Kradel D, Henzler DJ, Miller P, Key DW, Ruano M, Davison S. Summary of the 2001-02 Pennsylvania H7N2 low pathogenicity avian influenza outbreak in meat type chickens. *Avian Dis.* 2003;47(3 Suppl):812-6.

[16] Henzler DJ, Kradel DC, Davison S, Ziegler AF, Singletary D, DeBok P, Castro AE, Lu H, Eckroade R, Swayne D, Lagoda W, Schmucker B, Nesselrodt A. Epidemiology, production losses, and control measures associated with an outbreak of avian influenza subtype H7N2 in Pennsylvania (1996-98). *Avian Dis.* 2003;47(3 Suppl):1022-36.

[17] Lu H, Castro AE. Evaluation of the infectivity, length of infection, and immune response of a low-pathogenicity H7N2 avian influenza virus in specific-pathogen-free chickens. *Avian Dis.* 2004 Apr-Jun;48(2):263-70.

[18] Akey BL. Low-pathogenicity H7N2 avian influenza outbreak in Virgnia during 2002. *Avian Dis.* 2003;47(3 Suppl):1099-103.

[19] Tumpey TM, Kapczynski DR, Swayne DE. Comparative susceptibility of chickens and turkeys to avian influenza A H7N2 virus infection and protective efficacy of a commercial avian influenza H7N2 virus vaccine. *Avian Dis.* 2004 Jan-Mar;48(1):167-76.

[20] McQuiston JH, Garber LP, Porter-Spalding BA, Hahn JW, Pierson FW, Wainwright SH, Senne DA, Brignole TJ, Akey BL, Holt TJ. Evaluation of risk factors for the spread of low pathogenicity H7N2 avian influenza virus among commercial poultry farms. *J. Am. Vet. Med. Assoc.* 2005 Mar 1;226(5):767-72.

[21] Bowes VA. After the outbreak: how the British Columbia commercial poultry industry recovered after H7N3 HPAI. *Avian Dis.* 2007 Mar;51(1 Suppl):313-6.

[22] Skowronski DM, Li Y, Tweed SA, Tam TW, Petric M, David ST, Marra F, Bastien N, Lee SW, Krajden M, Brunham RC. Protective measures and human antibody response during an avian influenza H7N3 outbreak in poultry in British Columbia, Canada. *CMAJ.* 2007 Jan 2;176(1):47-53.

[23] Selleck PW, Arzey G, Kirkland PD, Reece RL, Gould AR, Daniels PW, Westbury HA. An outbreak of highly pathogenic avian influenza in Australia in 1997 caused by an H7N4 virus. *Avian Dis.* 2003;47(3 Suppl):806-11.

[24] Rohm C, Suss J, Pohle V, Webster RG. Different hemagglutinin cleavage site variants of H7N7 in an influenza outbreak in chickens in Leipzig, Germany. *Virology*. 1996 Apr 1;218(1):253-7.

[25] Elbers AR, Koch G, Bouma A. Performance of clinical signs in poultry for the detection of outbreaks during the avian influenza A (H7N7) epidemic in The Netherlands in 2003. *Avian Pathol*. 2005 Jun;34(3):181-7.

[26] Kwon YK, Lee YJ, Choi JG, Lee EK, Jeon WJ, Jeong OM, Kim MC, Joh SJ, Kwon JH, Kim JH. An outbreak of avian influenza subtype H9N8 among chickens in South Korea. *Avian Pathol*. 2006 Dec;35(6):443-7.

[27] Centers for Disease Control and Prevention (CDC), National Center for HIV/AIDS, Viral Hepatitis, STD, and TB Prevention. Prevention and control of tuberculosis in correctional and detention facilities: recommendations from CDC. Endorsed by the Advisory Council for the Elimination of Tuberculosis, the National Commission on Correctional Health Care, and the American Correctional Association. *MMWR Recomm. Rep.* 2006 Jul 7;55(RR-9):1-44.

[28] Brankston G, Gitterman L, Hirji Z, Lemieux C, Gardam M. Transmission of influenza A in human beings. *Lancet Infect. Dis.* 2007 Apr;7(4):257-65.

[29] Molinari JA. Infection control: its evolution to the current standard precautions. *J. Am. Dent. Assoc.* 2003 May;134(5):569-74.

[30] Garibaldi RA. Infection control in pulmonary and critical care medicine. *Semin. Respir. Infect.* 1999 Dec;14(4):372-82.

[31] Bagg J Common infectious diseases. Dent Clin North Am. 1996 Apr;40(2):385-93.

[32] Wright SA, Bieluch VM. Selected nosocomial viral infections. *Heart Lung*. 1993 Mar-Apr;22(2):183-7.

[33] Goldmann DA. Nosocomial viral infections: recent developments and new strategies. Eur *J. Clin. Microbiol. Infect. Dis.* 1989 Jan;8(1):75-81.

[34] Kappstein I, Daschner F. Hygienic and organizational precautions to prevent transmission of selected viral infections in hospitals] *Immun. Infekt.* 1988 Oct;16(5):192-6.

[35] Cates KL. Clinical considerations in the diagnosis of viral respiratory infections. *Diagn. Microbiol. Infect. Dis.* 1986 Mar;4(3 Suppl):23S-33S.

[36] Schunemann HJ, Hill SR, Kakad M, Bellamy R, Uyeki TM, Hayden FG, Yazdanpanah Y, Beigel J, Chotpitayasunondh T, Del Mar C, Farrar J, Tran TH, Ozbay B, Sugaya N, Fukuda K, Shindo N, Stockman L, Vist GE, Croisier A, Nagjdaliyev A, Roth C, Thomson G, Zucker H, Oxman AD; WHO Rapid Advice Guideline Panel on Avian Influenza.WHO Rapid Advice Guidelines for pharmacological management of sporadic human infection with avian influenza A (H5N1) virus. *Lancet Infect. Dis.* 2007 Jan;7(1):21-31.

[37] Lye DC, Nguyen DH, Giriputro S, Anekthananon T, Eraksoy H, Tambyah PA.Practical management of avian influenza in humans. *Singapore Med. J.* 2006 Jun;47(6):471-5.

[38] Lee VJ, Chen MI. Effectiveness of neuraminidase inhibitors for preventing staff absenteeism during pandemic influenza. *Emerg. Infect. Dis.* 2007 Mar;13(3):449-57.

[39] Gras-Masse H, Willand N. Neuraminidase inhibitors and risk of H5N1 influenza. *Ann. Pharm. Fr.* 2007 Jan;65(1):50-7.

[40] Hayden FG, Pavia AT. Antiviral management of seasonal and pandemic influenza. *J. Infect. Dis.* 2006 Nov 1;194 Suppl 2:S119-26.

[41] Singer AC, Nunn MA, Gould EA, Johnson AC. Potential risks associated with the proposed widespread use of Tamiflu. *Environ. Health Perspect.* 2007 Jan;115(1):102-6.

[42] Meyer KK, Beck WC. Gown-glove interface: a possible solution to the danger zone. *Infect. Control. Hosp. Epidemiol.* 1995 Aug;16(8):488-90.

[43] Medical waste disposal. Medical Waste Committee (WT-3). Technical Council Air and Waste Management Association. *Air Waste.* 1994 Oct;44(10):1176-9.

[44] Goldrick BA, Goetz AM. Pandemic influenza: what infection control professionals should know. *Am. J. Infect. Control.* 2007 Feb;35(1):7-13.

[45] Bird flu pandemic may not be certainty, but it's not too early to start preparing. *ED Manag.* 2005 Dec;17(12):133-6.

[46] Fica C A, Cifuentes D M, Ajenjo H MC, Delpiano M L, Febre V N, Medina L W, Parada E Y. Precautions in the care of patients hospitalized with H5N1 avian influenza. *Rev. Chilena Infectol.* 2006 Dec;23(4):290-6.

[47] Skowronski DM, Li Y, Tweed SA, Tam TW, Petric M, David ST, Marra F, Bastien N, Lee SW, Krajden M, Brunham RC. Protective measures and human antibody response during an avian influenza H7N3 outbreak in poultry in British Columbia, Canada. *CMAJ.* 2007 Jan 2;176(1):47-53.

[48] Tablan OC, Anderson LJ, Besser R, Bridges C, Hajjeh R; CDC; Healthcare Infection Control Practices Advisory Committee. Guidelines for preventing health-care--associated pneumonia, 2003: recommendations of CDC and the Healthcare Infection Control Practices Advisory Committee. *MMWR Recomm. Rep.* 2004 Mar 26;53(RR-3):1-36.

[49] Tellier R. Review of aerosol transmission of influenza A virus. *Emerg. Infect. Dis.* 2006 Nov;12(11):1657-62.

[50] Mardimae A, Slessarev M, Han J, Sasano H, Sasano N, Azami T, Fedorko L, Savage T, Fowler R, Fisher JA. Modified N95 mask delivers high inspired oxygen concentrations while effectively filtering aerosolized microparticles. *Ann. Emerg. Med.* 2006 Oct;48(4):391-9, 399.e1-2.

[51] Li Y, Wong T, Chung J, Guo YP, Hu JY, Guan YT, Yao L, Song QW, Newton E. In vivo protective performance of N95 respirator and surgical facemask. *Am. J. Ind. Med.* 2006 Dec;49(12):1056-65.

[52] Wiwanitkit V. N-95 face mask for prevention of bird flu virus: an appraisal of nanostructure and implication for infectious control. *Lung.* 2006 Nov-Dec;184(6):373-4.

[53] Kiselev OI, Sominina AA, Grinbaum EB. Influenza: current status and epidemiologic situation. *Vestn. Ross. Akad. Med. Nauk.* 1994;(9):3-7.

[54] Hosrtmann DM. Clinical virology. *Am. J. Med.* 1965 May;38:738-50.

[55] Thanawongnuwech R, Amonsin A, Tantilertcharoen R, Damrongwatanapokin S, Theamboonlers A, Payungporn S, Nanthapornphiphat K, Ratanamungklanon S, Tunak E, Songserm T, Vivatthanavanich V, Lekdumrongsak T, Kesdangsakonwut S, Tunhikorn S, Poovorawan Y. Probable tiger-to-tiger transmission of avian influenza H5N1. *Emerg. Infect. Dis.* 2005 May;11(5):699-701.

[56]   Amonsin A, Payungporn S, Theamboonlers A, Thanawongnuwech R, Suradhat S, Pariyothorn N, Tantilertcharoen R, Damrongwantanapokin S, Buranathai C, Chaisingh A, Songserm T, Poovorawan Y. Genetic characterization of H5N1 influenza A viruses isolated from zoo tigers in Thailand. *Virology.* 2006 Jan 20;344(2):480-91.

[57]   Amonsin A, Chutinimitkul S, Pariyothorn N, Songserm T, Damrongwantanapokin S, Puranaveja S, Jam-On R, Sae-Heng N, Payungporn S, Theamboonlers A, Chaisingh A, Tantilertcharoen R, Suradhat S, Thanawongnuwech R, Poovorawan Y. Genetic characterization of influenza A viruses (H5N1) isolated from 3rd wave of Thailand AI outbreaks. *Virus Res.* 2006 Dec;122(1-2):194-9.

[58]   Humphrey TJ. Contamination of egg shell and contents with Salmonella enteritidis: a review. *Int. J. Food Microbiol.* 1994 Jan;21(1-2):31-40.

[59]   Cox NA, Berrang ME, Cason JA. Salmonella penetration of egg shells and proliferation in broiler hatching eggs--a review. *Poult. Sci.* 2000 Nov;79(11):1571-4.

[60]   Savage CE, Jones RC. The survival of avian reoviruses on materials associated with the poultry house environment. *Avian Pathol.* 2003 Aug;32(4):419-25.

[61]   Little CL, Walsh S, Hucklesby L, Surman-Lee S, Pathak K, Hall Y, de Pinna E, Threlfall EJ, Maund A, Chan CH. Salmonella contamination in non-UK produced shell eggs on retail sale in some regions of England. *Euro Surveill.* 2006 Nov 23;11(11):E061123.4.

[62]   Board RG, Fuller R. Non-specific antimicrobial defences of the avian egg, embryo and neonate. *Biol. Rev. Camb. Philos. Soc.* 1974 Feb;49(1):15-49.

[63]   Maris P. Efficacy of disinfectants in contamination of eggs. *Ann. Rech. Vet.* 1986;17(2):123-8.

[64]   Whistler PE, Sheldon BW. Bactericidal activity, eggshell conductance, and hatchability effects of ozone versus formaldehyde disinfection. *Poult. Sci.* 1989 Aug;68(8):1074-7.

[65]   Khorol'skii LN, Khartsii KF. Disinfection of pheasant hatching eggs with formaldehyde fumes. *Veterinariia.* 1975 Apr;(4):28-9.

[66]   Maris P. Efficacy of disinfectants in contamination of eggs. *Ann. Rech. Vet.* 1986;17(2):123-8.

[67]   William JE. Effect of high-level formaldehyde fumigation on bacterial populations on the surface of chicken hatching eggs. *Avian Dis.* 1970 May;14(2):386-92.

[68]   Tan CK, Chen TW, Chan HL, Ng LS. A scanning and transmission electron microscopic study of the membranes of chicken egg. *Histol. Histopathol.* 1992 Jul;7(3):339-45.

[69]   Carrino DA, Dennis JE, Wu TM, Arias JL, Fernandez MS, Rodriguez JP, Fink DJ, Heuer AH, Caplan AI. The avian eggshell extracellular matrix as a model for biomineralization. *Connect. Tissue Res.* 1996;35(1-4):325-9.

[70]   Wiwanitkit V. Can avian bird flu virus pass through the eggshell? An appraisal and implications for infection control. *Am. J. Infect. Control.* 2007 Feb;35(1):71.

[71]   Avian flu. Available from http://thaigcd.ddc.moph.go.th/avianflu_FAQ_en.html.

[72]   Davis P. FDA researchers model virus transport through synthetic barriers. *SIAM News* 1998; 31: 1.

[73]   Influenza. Available from: http://users.rcn.com/jkimball.ma.ultranet /Biology Pages /I/Influenza.html.

[74] Bonchev N. Determination of fowl plague virus in the different parts of an infected incubated egg, *Izv. Akad. Nauk SSSR Biol.* 1950; 1: 199–204.

[75] Li Y, Lin Z, Shi J, Qi Q, Deng G, Li Z, Wang X, Tian G, Chen H. Detection of Hong Kong 97-like H5N1 influenza viruses from eggs of Vietnamese waterfowl. *Arch. Virol.* 2006 Aug;151(8):1615-24.

[76] Stromberg BE. Environmental factors influencing transmission.*Vet. Parasitol.* 1997 Nov;72(3-4):247-56

[77] Smith A, Rose SP, Wells RG, Pirgozliev V. The effect of changing the excreta moisture of caged laying hens on the excreta and microbial contamination of their egg shells. *Br. Poult. Sci.* 2000 May;41(2):168-73.

[78] Chotpitayasunondh T, Ungchusak K, Hanshaoworakul W, Chunsuthiwat S, Sawanpanyalert P, Kijphati R, Lochindarat S, Srisan P, Suwan P, Osotthanakorn Y, Anantasetagoon T, Kanjanawasri S, Tanupattarachai S, Weerakul J, Chaiwirattana R, Maneerattanaporn M, Poolsavathitikool R, Chokephaibulkit K, Apisarnthanarak A, Dowell SF. Human disease from influenza A (H5N1), Thailand, 2004. *Emerg. Infect. Dis.* 2005 Feb;11(2):201-9.

[79] Bublot M, Le Gros FX, Nieddu D, Pritchard N, Mickle TR, Swayne DE. Efficacy of two H5N9-inactivated vaccines against challenge with a recent H5N1 highly pathogenic avian influenza isolate from a chicken in Thailand. *Avian Dis.* 2007 Mar;51(1 Suppl):332-7.

[80] Tumpey TM, Suarez DL, Perkins LE, Senne DA, Lee JG, Lee YJ, Mo IP, Sung HW, Swayne DE. Characterization of a highly pathogenic H5N1 avian influenza A virus isolated from duck meat. *J. Virol.* 2002 Jun;76(12):6344-55.

[81] Tumpey TM, Suarez DL, Perkins LE, Senne DA, Lee J, Lee YJ, Mo IP, Sung HW, Swayne DE. Evaluation of a high-pathogenicity H5N1 avian influenza A virus isolated from duck meat. *Avian Dis.* 2003;47(3 Suppl):951-5.

[82] Lu X, Cho D, Hall H, Rowe T, Sung H, Kim W, Kang C, Mo I, Cox N, Klimov A, Katz J. Pathogenicity and antigenicity of a new influenza A (H5N1) virus isolated from duck meat. *J. Med. Virol.* 2003 Apr;69(4):553-9.

[83] Lu XH, Cho D, Hall H, Rowe T, Mo IP, Sung HW, Kim WJ, Kang C, Cox N, Klimov A, Katz JM. Pathogenesis of and immunity to a new influenza A (H5N1) virus isolated from duck meat. *Avian Dis.* 2003;47(3 Suppl):1135-40.

Chapter 9

Treatment of Human Bird Flu Infection

General Concept in Treatment for Influenza in Humans

Influenza is an important viral infection in humans. Preventive measures for influenza virus pneumonia center on limiting exposure of high-risk patients to active cases of influenza, administering annual vaccinations, and providing chemoprophylaxis [1]. Influenza is considered to be a self limited disease. Therapy for viral pneumonia is primarily supportive [1]. Symptomatic and supportive treatment can be used. Supportive therapy, including adequate tracheobronchial toilet, drainage of abscesses, oxygen inhalation, maintenance of adequate nutrition, and monitoring for super-infection; therapeutic effects may be life-saving in certain situations [2]. Symptom-based diagnosis remains the most commonly used strategy in clinical practice [3]. Antiviral therapy has been proposed for decades and can be used in selected cases [4]. The approval of the neuraminidase inhibitors, zanamivir and oseltamivir, remind healthcare providers of the difficulties in diagnosing and treating influenza [3]. These drugs have been shown to reduce the duration of symptoms of individuals infected with influenza when prescribed within the first 2 days of symptoms [3]. Cram et al. said that whether these innovative agents were cost effective, however, required a more detailed understanding of the benefits that these agents may offer above and beyond existing therapies [3]. Kashiwaki said that the anti-influenza agents were recommended to use within 48 hours after the onset of influenza because proliferation of influenza virus reached its peak after two days of the virus infection and the incubation period was only 24 hours [5]. Kashiwaki said that the patients beyond two days after the onset, patients should be treated by only anti-symptomatic therapies [5]. Jefferson et al. said that the use of amantadine and rimantadine should be discouraged because of the low effectiveness [6]. They noted that neuraminidase inhibitors should not be used in seasonal influenza control and should only be used in a serious epidemic or pandemic alongside other public-health measures [6]. Mossad quoted that anti-influenza drugs also had been shown to be useful prophylactically and to shorten the duration of illness by 1 or 2 days when started within 48 hours of symptom onset [7].

General Antiviral Drugs for Influenza

As previously mentioned, antiviral drugs for influenza is recommended in only some specific cases. Basically, there are two main groups of antiviral drugs for human influenza [8 - 17]. The first group is amantadines (amantadine and rimantadine) and the second group is neuraminidase inhibitors (oseltamivir and zanamivir). The development of the currently available classes of antivirals, the M2 proton channel inhibitors and the neuraminidase inhibitors, provides valuable perspectives relevant to the field of antiviral chemotherapy in general and insights into aspects of viral pathogenesis and antiviral resistance relevant specifically to influenza [17]. Amantadines group has a strong efficacy in destroying influenza type A virus but has no effect on influenza type B virus. This group is indicated for the patient aged above 1 year. The mechanism of action is direct binding to protein M2 on the surface of influenza virus. This binding mechanism can be the inhibition of cell invasion of the virus. Neuraminidase inhibitors can destroy both influenza type A and type B viruses. The mechanism of action is on viral neuraminidase enzyme. The inhibition of neuraminidase enzyme can cause the prevention of generation of new viruses from the viral infected cells. Consequently, the spread of the infection can be controlled. However, viruses resistant to the other anti-influenza drugs, neuraminidase inhibitors, have also been shown to emerge at a rate higher than previously thought [18]. In addition, several recent observations suggest that human-to-human transmission of variants resistant to neuraminidase inhibitors may have occurred, contrary to earlier predictions that such variants were much less likely to be transmitted [18]. For bird flu, amantadines group seems to be not effective since there are many reports on the mutation of M2 protein. For neuraminidase inhibitors, it is widely recommended as the antiviral drug of choice for bird flu.

Antiretroviral Drugs for Bird Flu

Since bird flu is a type of influenza, an oral disease, the main therapeutic option is combined supportive and symptomatic treatment. However, within a few years, advents on pharmaceutical technology led to many new antiviral drugs. For simple influenza, the need for specific antiviral drug treatment is low. Combined supportive and symptomatic treatment is sufficient. The use of an antibiotic drug is indicated in the case of superimposed infection, especially for community acquired pneumonia. Penicillin is indicated in those influenza infected cases with superimposed infections due to *Streptococcus pneumonia* [19 - 21].

Concerning bird flu, an antiviral drug is indicated. The use of an antiviral drug depends on availability of the drug in each setting [22 - 35]. Since most drugs are expensive, they seem to be unaffordable for these infected cares in the underdeveloped countries. The use of a drug relies on signs and symptoms of the patients, diagnostic procedures and decision making of the physicians in charge. As previously mentioned neuraminidase inhibitors is the drug of choice for treatment of bird flu in humans [36 – 37]. The general recommendation is prompt application of neuraminidase inhibitors. The golden period is within 48 hours because the peak of viral multiplication from infected cells is within 24-72 hours after the first signs and symptoms. A strong recommendation to treat H5N1 patients with oseltamivir was made in part because of the severity of the disease [37]. Similarly, strong recommendations were made to use neuraminidase inhibitors as chemoprophylaxis in high-risk exposure populations [37]. The details of important neuraminidase inhibitors will be hereby further discussed.

A. Oseltamivir [38 - 40]

Oseltamivir is the first drug that was introduced for treatment of human bird flu.

Pharmacologically, oseltamivir is the oral prodrug of GS4071, a selective inhibitor of influenza A and B viral neuraminidase [39 – 40]. After absorption from the gastrointestinal tract oseltamivir is efficiently converted to GS4071, which is maintained at high and sustained concentrations in plasma [38 – 40]. Based on studies in rats and ferrets, GS4071 appears to be effectively distributed to all tissues, including major sites of infection in the upper and lower respiratory tracts [38 – 40]. Oral oseltamivir was an effective treatment in naturally occurring influenza when administered within 36 hours of symptom onset, reducing both the duration and severity of symptoms and the incidence of secondary complications in influenza-infected patients enrolled in 2 large placebo-controlled, double-blind trials [38 – 40]. The major manufacturer of oseltamivir is the Roche company. The well-known trade name is "Tamiflu". Generally, there are two main forms of Tamiflu, capsule (75 mg) and powder. Tamiflu is well absorbed in the gastrointestinal tract and then metabolized at the liver into the active form, oseltamivir carboxylate. The oseltamivir carboxylate can actively affect the virus and has a half life about 6-10 hours. It is excreted via the kidneys; therefore, it is necessary to adapt dosage in cases with renal impairment. This drug is widely used for treatment and prevention of bird flu.

Studies in volunteers with experimental human influenza A or B showed that administration of oral oseltamivir 20 to 200 mg twice daily for 5 days reduced both the quantity and duration of viral shedding compared with placebo [38 - 40]. Subsequent assessment of the drug at a dosage of 75 mg twice daily for 5 days in otherwise healthy adults with naturally acquired febrile influenza showed that oseltamivir reduced the duration of the disease by up to 1.5 days and the severity of illness by up to 38% compared with placebo when initiated within 36 hours of symptom onset [38 – 40]. Hayden et al. performed a study to determine the safety, tolerability, and antiviral activity of oral neuraminidase inhibitor oseltamivir for prevention and the early treatment of influenza in experimentally infected humans [41]. Hayden et al. concluded that prophylaxis and early treatment with oral oseltamivir were both associated with significant antiviral and clinical effects in experimental human influenza [41]. Treanor et al. performed another study to evaluate the efficacy and safety of oseltamivir in the treatment of naturally acquired influenza infection [42]. Treanor et al. found that oral oseltamivir treatment reduced the duration and severity of acute influenza in healthy adults and might decrease the incidence of secondary complications [42]. In 2001, Li et al. performed another study to evaluate the efficacy and safety of oseltamivir in the treatment of naturally acquired influenza in China [43]. Li et al. concluded that adverse events reported were similar in oseltamivir and placebo group [43]. In this multicenter study, the main adverse events were gastrointestinal symptoms, headache, vertigo, and rashes [43]. Li et al. concluded that oseltamivir was effective and well tolerated in the treatment of early naturally acquired influenza [43]. Lin et al. performed a similar randomized controlled study of the efficacy and safety of oseltamivir in the treatment of influenza in a high risk population [44]. According to this study, Lin et al. suggested that oseltamivir was effective and well tolerated in patients with chronic respiratory or cardiac diseases [44]. Lin et al. said that oseltamivir could reduce the fever duration and severity of influenza symptoms, and could decrease the incidence of secondary complications and antibiotic use, while not increasing the total medical cost [44]. Deng et al. performed another multicenter study of efficacy and safety of oseltamivir in the treatment of suspected influenza patients [45]. Deng et al. suggested that Oseltamivir was effective and well tolerated in suspected influenza patients [45]. Deng et al. reported that oseltamivir could reduce the duration and severity of influenza symptoms and fever, and could decrease the incidence of suspected influenza in the contacted population using the antibiotic, with light side-effect [45]. Finally, Li et al. performed a double-blind, randomized, placebo-controlled multicenter study of oseltamivir phosphate for treatment of influenza infection in China [46]. Li et al. said that oseltamivir was effective and well tolerated as treatment of early naturally acquired influenza [46].

Concerning the pharmaceutical aspect of oseltamivir, this drug can be synthesized from natural Shikimic acid [47 – 55], which is an important intermediate in biosynthesis of many bio-substances including flavonoid, tannin and coumarin. The shikimic acid is firstly extracted from a plant namely Japanese star anise (*Illicium anisatum L.*) or shikimi. Shikimi is a small plant similar to Chinese star anise (*Illicium verum Hook. F.*). The useful paint is its fruit, which is eight star shape. It should be noted that although Japanese star anise is very similar to Chinese star anise in shape, the chemical properties are totally different. Chinese star anise is widely used as food additive; with well-known traditional name "Phoy-kuk" and can be applied as an important ingredient in classical Chinese medicine. While Japanese star anise cannot be used in its crude form due to the toxic components, anisatin, sikimitoxin and sikimin [56 – 57]. These phytotoxins cause concern, because of their bioactivation to reactive alkylating intermediates that are able to react with cellular macromolecules causing cellular toxicity, and, upon their reaction with DNA, genotoxicity resulting in tumors [56 – 57].

At present the two main indications for oseltamivir in human bird flu are a) any cases with a positive screening test for bird flu infection, and b) any medical personnel who has a history of contact with either human or animal bird flu infected cases and develop flu-like symptoms within a week. The dosage form of oseltamivir is 1 capsule bid for 5 days in adults. Dosage by body weight is presented in Table 1.

Although the effectiveness for treatment of human bird flu is confirmed, there are also many reports on the complications of usage or side effects of oseltamivir. The reported side effects include nausea, vomiting, anorexia, headache, and insomnia. Serious neuropsychosis is the most serious side effect [38 – 40, 58].

Table 1. Dosage of oseltamivir in pediatric cases

Body weight	Recommended dosage
< 15 kg	30 mg bid for 5 days
16-23 kg	45 mg bid for 5 days
24-40 kg	60 mg bid for 5 days
> 40 kg	75 mg (1 capsule) bid for 5 days

*The continuous monitoring of the side effect of oseltamivir is still needed.

For prevention, oseltamivir is proposed as a chemoprophylaxis [59]. Generally, in primary prevention, influenza vaccination is recommended for any medical personnel who have responsibilities for taking care of suspected patients with bird flu infection. In addition, these medical personnel are recommended to receive chemoprophylaxis by oseltamir. The recommended dosage form is one capsule per day for 30 days. This chemoprophylaxis is also suggested for any personnel who have to work in contact with dead animals suspected of having bird flu. Ward et al. said that if oseltamivir was included in a national or regional pandemic plan, stockpiling of the material, either in the form of capsules or the bulk active pharmaceutical ingredient would be necessary [59]. Ward et al. noted that there was no guarantee that an adequate supply of oseltamivir would be available in the absence of a stockpile [59].

The emerging problem of oseltamivir for treatment of human bird flu infection is the increasing of drug resistance [60]. A high rate of drug resistance in treatment of general influenza is reported. Recently, Smith et al. performed structural studies of the resistance of influenza virus neuramindase to inhibitors [61]. According to this study of Smith et al., the X-ray crystal structures of the complexes of BCX-1812 with the wild type and the two mutant neuraminidases were determined [61]. According to this work, a structural explanation of the mechanism of resistance of BCX-1812, relative to oseltamivir in particular, was provided [61].

In addition, there are reports of an oseltamivir-resistant strain of the virus in Vietnam. Close monitoring of the possible emergance and spread of a drug-resistant viral stain is a focus of present influenza research. Application of molecular epidemiology is needed in this situation.

B. Zanamivir [62 – 66]

Zanamivir is a new drug. It is in the form of diskhaler inhalation device. The main manufactures of Zanamivir is Glaxo-Wellcome company. The trade name is Relenza. After inhaling, the drug will directly enter into the respiratory tract, 10 % - 20 % into the lungs and the rest is left in the mouth and throat. The drug will be absorbed into blood circulation and 5 % to 15 % will be excreted via the urinary tract. Only 2 % of the administered drug can be detected in the blood stream. However, the drug level in the respiratory tract is sufficient for therapeutic effect, 1000 times the minimum, requirement of 50 % viral inhibition. This drug can be used for the patients over the age of 7 years. The recommended dosage is 2 blisters (1 blister = 5 mg) two times per day for 5 days. Drug administration should be started as early as possible. The golden period is within 2 days after the start of signs and symptoms. Because the dosage form of zanamivir is in a diskhaler, it is not as widely used as oseltamivir. However, the side effects of zanamivir are less commonly reported. The reported side effects include wheezing due to bronchus hyper-reactivity. In the cases with wheezing, bronchodilator in inhaler form must be administered. Due to this important side effect, zanamivir is contraindicated in cases with asthma or chronic obstructive lung disease. Ison et al. conducted a double-blind, randomized, placebo-controlled trial to assess the tolerability and efficacy of nebulized zanamivir in combination with rimantadine compared to rimantadine with nebulized saline for treating influenza in adults hospitalized with influenza [67]. Ison et al. quoted that nebulized zanamivir appeared to be well tolerated in the studied hospitalized population but further studies are needed to assess its efficacy [67]. Hayden et al. performed another study to assess the therapeutic activity of zanamivir in adults with acute influenza [68]. Hayden el al concluded that direct administration of a selective neuraminidase inhibitor, zanamivir, to the respiratory tract in adults with influenza A or B virus infections was safe and reduces symptoms if begun early [68]. Matsumoto et al. studied the therapeutic effects of zanamivir, a highly selective, potent and specific inhibitor of influenza A and B virus neuraminidases, in adult patients with acute influenza-like illness in Japan [69]. Matsumoto reported that topically administered zanamivir in adults was well tolerated and is effective in reducing the time for alleviation of influenza symptoms [69].

Govorkova et al. performed an interesting study aiming at comparison of efficacies of zanamivir, and oseltamivir against H5N1, H9N2, and other avian influenza viruses [70]. Govorkova et al. found that zanamivir had similar efficacy to oseltamivir against avian influenza viruses and might be of potential clinical use for treatment of emerging influenza viruses that may be transmitted from birds to humans [70]. In 2006, Li et al. synthesized new triazole-modified zanamivir analogues via click chemistry [71]. They reported that molecular modeling provided the information about the binding model between inhibitors and neuraminidase, which were in good agreement with inhibitory activities [71].

In addition to the basic antiviral drugs there are many trials on new developed drugs. These new drugs are the hope for effective treatment of H5N1 virus infection [72]. Examples of new drugs are cyclojzentone derivatives (BCX group) fludase, ampligen, peramivir and AV – 5706. These new drugs require many steps in pharmacological research before being launched for real use in the market.

1. Cyclopentane Derivatives

Cyclopentane derivatives have been widely tested in animal model studies. The important members of Cyclopentane derivatives are RWJ-270201, BCX – 1812, BCX – 1827, BCX – 1898 and BCX – 1923. In 2001, Smee et al. tested inhibition of viral cytopathic effect of RWJ-270201 [73].

Smee et al. reported that exposure of cells to RWJ-270201 caused most of the virus to remain cell associated, with extracellular virus decreasing in a concentration-dependent manner and this was consistent with its effect as a neuraminidase inhibitor [73]. Smee et al.

concluded that RWJ-270201 showed promise in the treatment of human influenza virus infections [73].

2. Fludase

Fludase is a new diskhaler form antiviral drug. It was developed by the San Diego Firm NexBio. This drug has not yet been launched (2007).

3. Ampligen [74]

Ampligen is developed by Hemisphrex Biopharma of Philadelphia. It is a drug designed to increase immune response to oseltinavir, zanamivir, and influenza vaccine. Ampligen is also applied for many other viral infections.

4. Peramivir [75 – 80]

Peramivir is developed by AV 1 Biopharm, Portland. This is a new drug designed to target at the viral nucleic acid to disturb the viral multiplication. Peramivir is a cyclopentane derivative (BCX-1812, RWJ-270201). In Phase I studies, peramivir was well-tolerated, with single or multiple oral doses up to 800 mg/kg/day evaluated. In clinical trials with patients experimentally infected with influenza A or B viruses, oral treatment with peramivir significantly reduced nasal wash virus titres with no adverse effects [77]. Based on the high selectivity and efficacy of peramivir against both type A and B influenza strains in preclinical studies as well as murine pharmacodynamic studies supporting the potential for once-daily administration, clinical trials were initiated in order to determine the tolerability and antiviral activity of peramivir in humans [75]. To date, clinical studies have indicated that peramivir is well tolerated and has antiviral activity in human experimental influenza models [75]. The in vitro potency of peramivir appears to be greater than either zanamivir or oseltamivir carboxylate based on the generally lower EC(50) values seen using peramivir in studies run in parallel with each compound [75 - 80]. A pharmacokinetic study of this compound in influenza virus-infected mice indicates once-, twice- or thrice-daily oral dosing is equal in efficacy; once-daily dosing has been recommended in influenza therapy [75 – 80]. Although peramivir is a rather new drug, resistance has already been reported since 2007 [81].

References

[1]   Chien JW, Johnson JL. Viral pneumonias. Epidemic respiratory viruses. *Postgrad. Med.* 2000 Mar;107(3):41-2, 45-7, 51-2.
[2]   Tecson F, Louria DB. Infectious pneumonias: a review. *J. Fam. Pract.* 1977 Feb;4(2):201-9.

[3]   Cram P, Blitz SG, Monto A, Fendrick AM. Influenza. Cost of illness and considerations in the economic evaluation of new and emerging therapies. *Pharmacoeconomics.* 2001;19(3):223-30.

[4]   Bauer DJ. Antiviral chemotherapy. *Mod Trends Med Virol.* 1967;1(0):49-76.

[5]   Kashiwagi S. Criteria for the use of anti-influenza agents. *Nippon Rinsho.* 2003 Nov;61(11):1963-6.

[6]   Jefferson T, Demicheli V, Rivetti D, Jones M, Di Pietrantonj C, Rivetti A. Antivirals for influenza in healthy adults: systematic review. *Lancet.* 2006 Jan 28;367(9507):303-13.

[7]   Mossad SB. Prophylactic and symptomatic treatment of influenza. Current and developing options. *Postgrad. Med.* 2001 Jan;109(1):97-105

[8]   Turkulov V, Madle-Samardzija N. Influenza--always present among us. *Med. Pregl.* 2000 Mar-Apr;53(3-4):154-8.

[9]   Saito R, Suzuki H. Antiviral agents for influenza. *Nippon Rinsho.* 2007 Feb 28;65 Suppl 2 Pt. 1:401-6.

[10] Lynch JP 3rd, Walsh EE. Influenza: evolving strategies in treatment and prevention. *Semin. Respir. Crit. Care Med.* 2007 Apr;28(2):144-58.

[11] American Academy of Pediatrics Committee on Infectious Diseases. Antiviral therapy and prophylaxis for influenza in children. *Pediatrics.* 2007 Apr;119(4):852-60.

[12] De Clercq E. Antiviral agents active against influenza A viruses. *Nat. Rev. Drug. Discov.* 2006 Dec;5(12):1015-25.

[13] Stock I. Human influenza. *Med. Monatsschr. Pharm.* 2006 Oct;29(10):360-8; quiz 369-70.

[14] Antiviral drugs prophylaxis and treatment of influenza. *Med. Lett. Drugs Ther.* 2006 Oct 23;48(1246):87-8.

[15] Sugaya N. Treatment of influenza virus infection with anti-virals. *Nippon Rinsho.* 2006 Oct;64(10):1840-4.

[16] Mitamura K, Sugaya N. Diagnosis and Treatment of influenza--clinical investigation on viral shedding in children with influenza. *Uirusu.* 2006 Jun;56(1):109-16.

[17] Hayden FG. Antivirals for influenza: historical perspectives and lessons learned. *Antiviral Res.* 2006 Sep;71(2-3):372-8.

[18] Hatakeyama S, Kawaoka Y. The molecular basis of resistance to anti-influenza drugs. *Nippon Rinsho.* 2006 Oct;64(10):1845-52.

[19] Grant CC, Ingram RJ. Outpatient treatment of pneumonia. *N. Z. Med. J.* 2000 Feb 25;113(1104):58-62.

[20] Leedom JM. Pneumonia. Patient profiles, choice of empiric therapy, and the place of third-generation cephalosporins. *Diagn. Microbiol. Infect. Dis.* 1992 Jan;15(1):57-65.

[21] Hedlund J, Stralin K, Ortqvist A, Holmberg H; Community-Acquired Pneumonia Working Group of the Swedish Society of Infectious Diseases. Swedish guidelines for the management of community-acquired pneumonia in immunocompetent adults. *Scand. J. Infect. Dis.* 2005;37(11-12):791-805.

[22] Kashiwagi S. Threat from newly emerging influenza. *Nippon Naika Gakkai Zasshi.* 2007 Apr 10;96(4):811-6.

[23] Rajagopal S, Treanor J. Pandemic (avian) influenza. *Semin. Respir. Crit. Care Med.* 2007 Apr;28(2):159-70.

[24] Krau SD, Parsons LC. Avian influenza: are we ready? *Crit. Care Nurs. Clin. North Am.* 2007 Mar;19(1):107-13.

[25] Hoheisel G, Luk WK, Winkler J, Wirtz H, Gillissen A, Hui DS, Liebert UG. Avian influenza and the Severe Acute Respiratory Syndrome (SARS) - experiences and perspectives. *Pneumologie.* 2007 Jan;61(1):41-5.

[26] Hurtado TR. Human influenza A (H5N1): a brief review and recommendations for travelers. *Wilderness Environ. Med.* 2006 Winter;17(4):276-81.

[27] Thomas JK, Noppenberger J. Avian influenza: a review. *Am. J. Health Syst. Pharm.* 2007 Jan 15;64(2):149-65.

[28] Cox MM. Pandemic influenza: overview of vaccines and antiviral drugs. *Yale J. Biol. Med.* 2005 Oct;78(5):321-8.

[29] Harrod ME, Emery S, Dwyer DE. Antivirals in the management of an influenza pandemic. *Med .J. Aust.* 2006 Nov 20;185(10 Suppl):S58-61.

[30] Lye DC, Nguyen DH, Giriputro S, Anekthananon T, Eraksoy H, Tambyah PA. Practical management of avian influenza in humans. Singapore *Med. J.* 2006 Jun;47(6):471-5.

[31] Saeed AA, Hussein MF. Avian influenza. *Saudi Med. J.* 2006 May;27(5):585-95.

[32] Stephenson I, Democratis J. Influenza: current threat from avian influenza. *Br. Med. Bull.* 2006 May 1;75-76:63-80.

[33] Garcia-Garcia J, Ramos C. Influenza, an existing public health problem. *Salud. Publica. Mex.* 2006 May-Jun;48(3):244-67.

[34] Campbell S. Avian influenza: are you prepared? *Nurs Stand.* 2006 Oct 11-17;21(5): 51-6.

[35] Juckett G. Avian influenza: preparing for a pandemic. *Am. Fam. Physician.* 2006 Sep 1;74(5):783-90.

[36] Gras-Masse H, Willand N. Neuraminidase inhibitors and risk of H5N1 influenza. *Ann. Pharm. Fr.* 2007 Jan;65(1):50-7.

[37] Schunemann HJ, Hill SR, Kakad M, Bellamy R, Uyeki TM, Hayden FG, Yazdanpanah Y, Beigel J, Chotpitayasunondh T, Del Mar C, Farrar J, Tran TH, Ozbay B, Sugaya N, Fukuda K, Shindo N, Stockman L, Vist GE, Croisier A, Nagjdaliyev A, Roth C, Thomson G, Zucker H, Oxman AD; WHO Rapid Advice Guideline Panel on Avian Influenza. WHO Rapid Advice Guidelines for pharmacological management of sporadic human infection with avian influenza A (H5N1) virus. *Lancet Infect. Dis.* 2007 Jan;7(1):21-31.

[38] Bardsley-Elliot A, Noble S. Oseltamivir. *Drugs.* 1999 Nov;58(5):851-60.

[39] McClellan K, Perry CM. Oseltamivir: a review of its use in influenza. *Drugs.* 2001;61(2):263-83.

[40] McNicholl IR, McNicholl JJ. Neuraminidase inhibitors: zanamivir and oseltamivir. *Ann. Pharmacother..* 2001 Jan;35(1):57-70.

[41] Hayden FG, Treanor JJ, Fritz RS, Lobo M, Betts RF, Miller M, Kinnersley N, Mills RG, Ward P, Straus SE. Use of the oral neuraminidase inhibitor oseltamivir in

experimental human influenza: randomized controlled trials for prevention and treatment. *JAMA*. 1999 Oct 6;282(13):1240-6.

[42] Treanor JJ, Hayden FG, Vrooman PS, Barbarash R, Bettis R, Riff D, Singh S, Kinnersley N, Ward P, Mills RG. Efficacy and safety of the oral neuraminidase inhibitor oseltamivir in treating acute influenza: a randomized controlled trial. US Oral Neuraminidase Study Group. *JAMA*. 2000 Feb 23;283(8):1016-24.

[43] Li L, Cai B, Wang M, Zhu Y. A multicenter study of efficacy and safety of oseltamivir in treatment of naturally acquired influenza. *Zhonghua Nei Ke Za Zhi*. 2001 Dec;40(12):838-42.

[44] Lin JT, Yu XZ, Cui DJ, Chen XY, Zhu JH, Wang YZ, Wu XD, Gao H, Huo ZL, Zhu SH, Hu SL, Wang AX. A multicenter randomized controlled study of the efficacy and safety of oseltamivir in the treatment of influenza in a high risk population. *Zhonghua Jie He He Hu Xi Za Zhi*. 2004 Jul;27(7):455-9.

[45] Deng WW, Li QY, Zhong NS; "Oseltamivir in the treatment of suspected influenza patients" Study Group. A multicenter study of efficacy and safety of oseltamivir in the treatment of suspected influenza patients. *Zhonghua Yi Xue Za Zhi*. 2004 Dec 17;84(24):2132-6.

[46] Li L, Cai B, Wang M, Zhu Y. A double-blind, randomized, placebo-controlled multicenter study of oseltamivir phosphate for treatment of influenza infection in China. *Chin. Med. J. (Engl)*. 2003 Jan;116(1):44-8.

[47] Knaggs AR. The biosynthesis of shikimate metabolites. *Nat. Prod. Rep.* 2003 Feb;20(1):119-36.

[48] Knaggs AR. The biosynthesis of shikimate metabolites. *Nat. Prod. Rep.* 2001 Jun;18(3):334-55.

[49] Dewick PM. The biosynthesis of shikimate metabolites. Nat *Prod Rep.* 1998 Feb;15(1):17-58.

[50] Dewick PM. The biosynthesis of shikimate metabolites. *Nat. Prod. Rep.* 1995 Dec;12(6):579-607.

[51] Dewick PM. The biosynthesis of shikimate metabolites. *Nat. Prod. Rep.* 1993 Jun;10(3):233-63.

[52] Dewick PM. The biosynthesis of shikimate metabolites. *Nat. Prod. Rep.* 1992 Apr;9(2):153-81.

[53] Dewick PM. The biosynthesis of shikimate metabolites. Nat *Prod Rep.* 1991 Apr;8(2):149-70.

[54] Dewick PM. The biosynthesis of shikimate metabolites. *Nat. Prod. Rep.* 1990 Jun;7(3):165-89.

[55] Dewick PM. The biosynthesis of shikimate metabolites. *Nat. Prod. Rep.* 1989 Jun;6(3):263-90.

[56] Fujii M. Plant toxicity-coriamyrtin, anisatin, cicutoxin. *Ryoikibetsu Shokogun Shirizu*. 1999;(27 Pt 2):682-4.

[57] Rietjens IM, Martena MJ, Boersma MG, Spiegelenberg W, Alink GM. Molecular mechanisms of toxicity of important food-borne phytotoxins. *Mol. Nutr. Food Res.* 2005 Feb;49(2):131-58.

[58] Jones M, Del Mar C. Safety of neuraminidase inhibitors for influenza. *Expert Opin. Drug Saf.* 2006 Sep;5(5):603-8.

[59] Ward P, Small I, Smith J, Suter P, Dutkowski R. Oseltamivir (Tamiflu) and its potential for use in the event of an influenza pandemic. *J. Antimicrob. Chemother..* 2005 Feb;55 Suppl. 1:i5-i21.

[60] Oxford JS, Mann A, Lambkin R. A designer drug against influenza: the NA inhibitor oseltamivir (Tamiflu). *Expert Rev. Anti Infect. Ther.* 2003 Aug;1(2):337-42.

[61] Smith BJ, McKimm-Breshkin JL, McDonald M, Fernley RT, Varghese JN, Colman PM. Structural studies of the resistance of influenza virus neuramindase to inhibitors. *J. Med. Chem.* 2002 May 23;45(11):2207-12.

[62] Alymova IV, Taylor G, Portner A. Neuraminidase inhibitors as antiviral agents. *Curr. Drug. Targets Infect. Disord.* 2005 Dec;5(4):401-9.

[63] Mayor S. Review says oseltamivir and zanamivir should be kept for epidemics of flu. *BMJ.* 2006 Jan 28;332(7535):196.

[64] Oxford JS. Zanamivir (Glaxo Wellcome). *IDrugs.* 2000 Apr;3(4):447-59.

[65] Kashiwagi S. Zanamivir, oseltamivir. *Nippon Rinsho.* 2004 Dec;62 Suppl 12:445-7.

[66] Cheer SM, Wagstaff AJ. Spotlight on zanamivir in influenza. *Am. J. Respir. Med.* 2002;1(2):147-52.

[67] Ison MG, Gnann JW Jr, Nagy-Agren S, Treannor J, Paya C, Steigbigel R, Elliott M, Weiss HL, Hayden FG; NIAID Collaborative Antiviral Study Group. Safety and efficacy of nebulized zanamivir in hospitalized patients with serious influenza. *Antivir. Ther.* 2003 Jun;8(3):183-90.

[68] Hayden FG, Osterhaus AD, Treanor JJ, Fleming DM, Aoki FY, Nicholson KG, Bohnen AM, Hirst HM, Keene O, Wightman K. Efficacy and safety of the neuraminidase inhibitor zanamivir in the treatment of influenzavirus infections. GG167 *Influenza Study Group. N. Engl. J. Med.* 1997 Sep 25;337(13):874-80.

[69] Matsumoto K, Ogawa N, Nerome K, Numazaki Y, Kawakami Y, Shirato K, Arakawa M, Kudoh S, Shimokata K, Nakajima S, Yamakido M, Kashiwagi S, Nagatake T. Safety and efficacy of the neuraminidase inhibitor zanamivir in treating influenza virus infection in adults: results from Japan. GG167 Group. *Antivir. Ther..* 1999;4(2):61-8.

[70] Govorkova EA, Leneva IA, Goloubeva OG, Bush K, Webster RG. Comparison of efficacies of RWJ-270201, zanamivir, and oseltamivir against H5N1, H9N2, and other avian influenza viruses. *Antimicrob. Agents Chemother..* 2001 Oct;45(10):2723-32.

[71] Li J, Zheng M, Tang W, He PL, Zhu W, Li T, Zuo JP, Liu H, Jiang H. Syntheses of triazole-modified zanamivir analogues via click chemistry and anti-AIV activities. *Bioorg. Med. Chem. Lett.* 2006 Oct 1;16(19):5009-13.

[72] Wiwanitkit V. Current research on drugs and vaccines for fighting bird flu. *Trans. R. Soc. Trop. Med. Hyg.* 2007 Jul 24;

[73] Smee DF, Huffman JH, Morrison AC, Barnard DL, Sidwell RW. Cyclopentane neuraminidase inhibitors with potent in vitro anti-influenza virus activities. *Antimicrob. Agents Chemother.* 2001 Mar;45(3):743-8.

[74] Brodsky I, Strayer DR. Therapeutic potential of Ampligen. *Am. Fam. Physician.* 1987 Oct;36(4):253-6.

[75] Young D, Fowler C, Bush K. RWJ-270201 (BCX-1812): a novel neuraminidase inhibitor for influenza. *Philos. Trans. R. Soc. Lond B. Biol Sci.* 2001 Dec 29;356(1416):1905-13.

[76] Barnard DL. RWJ-270201 BioCryst Pharmaceuticals/Johnson and Johnson. *Curr. Opin. Investig. Drugs.* 2000 Dec;1(4):421-4.

[77] Sidwell RW, Smee DF. Peramivir (BCX-1812, RWJ-270201): potential new therapy for influenza. *Expert. Opin. Investig. Drugs.* 2002 Jun;11(6):859-69.

[78] Reina J. Peramivir. A new and potent neuraminidase inhibitor for the treatment of influenza. *Rev. Esp. Quimioter.* 2006 Dec;19(4):317-22.

[79] Viegas TX, Goodin RR, Winkle LV, Hawthorne RB. Physicochemical properties of the potent influenza neuraminidase inhibitor, peramivir (BCX-1812). *J. Pharm. Biomed. Anal.* 2007 Jul 10;

[80] Babu YS, Chand P, Bantia S, Kotian P, Dehghani A, El-Kattan Y, Lin TH, Hutchison TL, Elliott AJ, Parker CD, Ananth SL, Horn LL, Laver GW, Montgomery JA. BCX-1812 (RWJ-270201): discovery of a novel, highly potent, orally active, and selective influenza neuraminidase inhibitor through structure-based drug design. *J. Med. Chem.* 2000 Sep 21;43(19):3482-6.

[81] Baz M, Abed Y, Boivin G. Characterization of drug-resistant recombinant influenza A/H1N1 viruses selected in vitro with peramivir and zanamivir. *Antiviral. Res.* 2007 May;74(2):159-62.

Chapter 10

Prevention of Bird Flu Infection

Introduction

During the last decade, the number of reported outbreaks caused by highly pathogenic avian influenza (HPAI) in domestic poultry has drastically increased [1]. At the same time, low pathogenic avian influenza (LPAI) strains, such as H9N2 in many parts of the Middle East and Asia and H6N2 in live bird markets in California, have become endemic [1]. Since 1997, an influenza virus of avian origin has appeared regularly in humans causing severe respiratory infections leading to death in half cases [2]. This Influenza A (H5N I) virus which is at the origin of this illness circulates in wild birds and in domestic birds [2]. A million poultry have been regularly infected or slaughtered on 3 continents: Asia, Africa and Europe [2]. An influenza pandemic is believed to be imminent. The only questions are what will be the causative agent and when will it happen [3].

Preventive medicine can be applied for the prevention of bird flu infection [4]. Primary and secondary prevention are useful. Primary prevention includes health education and vaccination. Secondary prevention includes early diagnosis and prompt treatment. In this chapter, the author will discuss the preventive medicine for bird flu infection.

Health Education for Bird Flu Infection

Health education is a core for primary prevention of infectious disease. A program that aims to assist healthcare workers to prepare, both in their professional and personal life, for a possible influenza pandemic is necessary [5]. The most effective way to reduce the spread of the virus is with good infection-control practices and social distancing [6]. Infection-control practices include the use of personal protective equipment, hand hygiene, respiratory hygiene and cough etiquette [6]. Infected people should be isolated and spatial separation observed in common areas where infected people may be present [6]. To derive the mentioned behaviors, health education is needed. Australian pandemic plans acknowledge a role for general practice, but there are few published data addressing the issues that general practitioners and their practices will face in dealing with such a crisis [7]. The outcome will revolve around preparation in three key areas: definition of the role of general practice within a broad primary care pandemic response, and adequate preparation within general practices so they can play that role well [7]. Given the current situation, it is imperative that close collaboration is sought and achieved by public health officials involved in the veterinary and medical aspects of the disease [8].

To make a favorable practice, good knowledge and attitude are necessary. There are some recent knowledge-attitude-practice (KAP) survey studies on influenza. Willis and Wortley confirmed the importance of comprehensive approaches that combined education and convenience, and suggested that emphasizing the rationale for health care worker vaccination might contribute to increasing vaccination rates [9]. A study was designed by Esposito et al. to evaluate compliance with recommendations concerning the use of influenza vaccine by practitioners for their pregnant and pediatric patients [10]. The results clearly showed that only a marginal number of the health care workers recommended vaccine use for pregnant women and healthy young children [10]. Moreover, all of the health care workers were seriously deficient in terms of their general knowledge of influenza prevention, and their own personal vaccination coverage was low [10]. Daley et al. performed another survey on parents from metropolitan Denver, Colorado, about influenza vaccination [11]. According to this work, parents of young children hold a number of misperceptions about influenza disease and vaccination [11]. Despite this, high immunization rates are achievable in this population [11]. Kristiansen et al. performed another interesting study on perception of risk and individual precautions in a general population in Norway [12]. The main outcome measures were answers to questions about a potential pandemic ("serious influenza epidemic"): statements about personal precautions including stockpiling the anti-influenza drug Tamiflu, the perceived number of fatalities, the perceived effects of Tamilfu, the sources of information about influenza and trust in public information [12]. According to this work, considerable proportions of people seem to consider the mortality risk during a pandemic less than health authorities do [12]. Most people seem to be prepared to take some, but not especially disruptive, precautions [12]. Al-Shehri et al. recently identified knowledge and concerns about avian influenza among secondary school students in Taif, Saudi Arabia [13]. According to this study, knowledge scores were significantly related to socioeconomic indicators and approximately 70% of the participants reported that media (television or radio) was the source of their information [13]. Of interest, 65.4% of the participants said they expected there to be cases of avian influenza in Saudi Arabia in 2006 [13]. Al-Shehri et al. proposed that effective school health education programs should be implemented in order to prepare the community to deal with this possible important threat [13]. Al-Turki studied awareness of avian influenza among attendees of a primary healthcare clinic in Riyadh and reported that health education was still needed to increase correct knowledge among the general population [14]. Lau et al. recently performed a random, anonymous, cross-sectional telephone survey on anticipated and current preventive behaviors in response to an anticipated human-to-human H5N1 epidemic in the Hong Kong Chinese general population [15]. Lau et al. concluded that the public in Hong Kong was likely to adopt preventive measures that might help contain the spread of the virus in the community in the event of a human-to-human H5N1 outbreak [15]. Lau et al. also reported that panic and interruption of daily routines might occur in the event of a human avian influenza outbreak [16]. Lau et al.

noted that dissemination of accurate, timely information would reduce unnecessary distress and unwanted behaviors [16]. Fielding et al. performed a telephone survey of 986 Hong Kong households to determine exposure and risk perception of avian influenza from live chicken sales [17]. According to this study, age, avian influenza contagion worries, husbandry threat, avian influenza threat, and avian influenza anxiety predicted perceived sickness risk [17]. High population exposures to live chickens and low perceived risk were potentially important health threats in avian influenza [17]. Leggat et al. performed a study on hostellers' knowledge of transmission and prevention of avian influenza when travelling abroad [18]. According to this work, hostellers attending the travelers' information night in Australia reported having moderate concern about avian influenza [18]. They also had a variable knowledge of the sources of infection of avian influenza [18]. Leggat et al. proposed that although hostellers responded positively to hand-washing advice provided in the travel health lecture, reinforcement of other possible measures to prevent avian influenza, particularly the possible role of antiviral drugs, might be needed [19]. Abbate et al. performed a KAP survey of avian influenza among poultry workers in Italy [19]. Abbate et al. noted that health education in this area was still needed [19].

Avian Flu Vaccination for Birds

Recent outbreaks of highly pathogenic avian influenza A virus infections in poultry and humans through direct contact with infected birds have raised concerns that a new influenza pandemic might occur in the near future [20 – 23]. Effective vaccines against H5N1 virus are, therefore, urgently needed [20 – 23]. Vaccine for bird flu in animals has a long history. Bird flu vaccination is widely used in veterinarian medicine. There are two types of vaccine, live and non-live vaccine. Live vaccine contains a genetically modified virus that can further multiply in vivo in birds [20 - 23]. There are pro and con aspects for avian flu vaccine. The advantage of vaccination in birds is prevention of pandemic outbreak among birds. The vaccine can decrease morbidity and mortality in birds. In addition, the vaccinated animals excrete lower virus than that of non vaccinated animals, therefore, the transmission rate can be decreased. The application of control policies, ranging from stamping out to emergency and prophylactic vaccination, are discussed on the basis of data generated from recent outbreaks, in the light of new regulations and also in view of the maintenance of animal welfare [24]. Poultry veterinarians working for the industry or for the public sector represent the first line of defense against the pandemic threat and for the prevention and control of this infection in poultry and in wild birds [24]. However, given the current situation, it is imperative that close collaboration is sought and achieved by health officials involved in the veterinary, agricultural and medical aspects of the disease [25]. Effective vaccines against H5N1 virus are needed [26]. Subtype H5 AI vaccine has been shown to provide protection against heterologous H5 strains with 89.4% or greater hemagglutinin deduced amino acid sequence similarity and isolated over decades [27]. Currently, inactivated whole AI virus vaccines and a fowl pox-vectored vaccine with avian influenza H5 hemagglutinin gene insert are used commercially in various countries of the world [27]. Reverse-genetics-based inactivated vaccines have been prepared according to World Health Organization (WHO) recommendations and are now undergoing clinical evaluation in several countries [26]. Of several new avian influenza vaccine, the avian influenza vaccines designated TROVAC-AIV H5 (TROVAC-H5) contains a live recombinant fowlpox rec. (FP) recombinant (recFP), expressing the hemagglutinin gene of an avian influenza H5 subtype isolate [28]. This recombinant vaccine was granted a license in the United States for emergency use in 1998 and full registration in Mexico, Guatemala, and El Salvador where over 2 billion doses have been administered [28]. One injection of TROVAC-H5 protects chickens against avian influenza-induced mortality and morbidity for at least 20 weeks, and significantly decreases shedding after challenge with a wide panel of H5-subtype avian influenza strains, regardless of neuraminidase subtype [28]. In 2007, Bublot et al. evaluated the efficacy of rFP-AIV-H5 against escalating doses of highly pathogenic avian influenza (HPAI) H5N1 A/chicken/ SouthKorea/ES/03 isolate and against the HPAI H5N1 A/chicken/Vietnam/0008/2004 isolate [29]. Bublot et al. confirmed the excellent level of protection induced by rFP-AIV-H5 in SPF chickens against two recent Asian HPAI H5N1 isolates [29]. Karaca et al. performed another study to evaluate immunogenicity of AIV-H5 in cats [30]. According to this study, Karaca et al. concluded that the vaccine and other poxvirus-vectored vaccines might be of value for the prophylaxis of avian influenza virus-associated morbidity and mortality in mammals [30]. According to another study by Steensels et al., the efficacy of an inactivated vaccine containing the Eurasian isolate A/chicken/Italy/22A/98 H5N9 (H5N9-It) was compared with that of the rFP-AIV-H5 vaccine against an H5N1 HPAI challenge [31]. According to this study, the inactivated vaccine induced hemagglutination inhibition titers that were boosted after the second administration [31]. The rFP-AIV-H5-induced HI titers were lower, most probably because the fowlpox vector does not replicate in ducks [31]. Altogether, these results indicate that significant protection from clinical signs and reduction in virus shedding may be achieved in ducks with conventional inactivated or fowlpox-vectored vaccine as compared with nonvaccinated challenged control birds [31]. Bublot el al performed another interesting study to compare the efficacy of two avian influenza H5-inactivated vaccines containing either an American (A/turkey/Wisconsin/68 H5N9; H5N9-WI) or a Eurasian isolate (H5N9-It) in Thailand [32]. Bublot et al. indicated that both vaccines protected very well against morbidity and mortality and reduced or prevented shedding induced by direct or contact exposure to Asian H5N1 HPAI virus [32].

In addition to vector vaccine, there are also other new vaccines [27]. DNA vaccine is another new type. Laddy et al. proposed a novel consensus-based approach to vaccine development, employing a DNA vaccine strategy that could provide more highly cross-reactive cellular immunity against lethal influenza infection [33]. Lee et al. noted that DNA vaccination provided a safer alternative for the production of hemagglutination-specific antibodies, since it was produced without the use of live virus [34]. Kodihalli et al. performed a study to assess cross-protection among lethal H5N2 influenza viruses induced by DNA vaccine to the hemagglutinin [35]. The absence of detectable antibody titers after primary immunization, together with the rapid appearance of high titers immediately after challenge, implicated efficient B-cell priming as the principal mechanism of DNA-mediated immune protection [35]. Kodihalli et al. suggested that the efficacy of hemagglutination-DNA influenza virus vaccine in mice extended to chickens and probably to other avian species as well [35]. Le Gall-Recule et al. initiated studies targeting prevention of H7 infection through

DNA vaccines encoding H7 and M1 viral proteins from an Italian H7N1 LPAI virus isolated from poultry in 1999 [36]. According to this work, after the homologous challenge, chickens of every vaccinated group displayed a significant decrease in cloacal shedding, whereas tracheal shedding was not significantly reduced in the protein/protein group [36]. After the heterologous challenge, only the DNA/DNA group showed a nonsignificant decrease in tracheal shedding [36]. According to these two trials, prime-boost DNA/protein vaccination appeared to be more advantageous [36]. Subunit protein vaccine is another vaccine type. In development, both hemagglutinin and neuraminidase are the focus. Style et al. found that vaccination with A/Pheasant/Maryland /4457/93 (Ph/MD) rN2 protein produced significantly higher levels of neuraminidase - inhibition activity and 88% protection from HPAI H5N2 challenge than vaccination with Ph/MD N2 DNA [37]. The fraction nucleoprotein/hemagglutinin obtained from n-octyl-beta-D-glucopyranoside-treated influenza A H5N2 virus is highly enriched for NP with residual hemagglutinin [38]. This potent immunostimulating complex can induce the production of high antibody titres in turkeys [38]. The nucleoprotein/hemagglutinin preparation is found to protect turkeys from both homologous and heterologous challenge infection as shown by reduced viral titers in the lung and trachea of vaccinated turkeys [38]. From the perspective of human health, it is essential to eradicate the virus from poultry; however, the large number of small-holdings with poultry, the lack of control experience and resources, and the international scale of transmission and infection make rapid control and long-term prevention of recurrence extremely difficult [39]. Ellis et al. reported their experience on how vaccination of chickens against H5N1 avian influenza in the face of an outbreak interrupts virus transmission [40]. They concluded that H5 vaccine could interrupt virus transmission in a field setting [40].

Considering the disadvantage, the efficacy of the vaccine is not 100 % therefore, infection can still occur. These vaccinated but infected birds can be the silent carrier and transmit to the environment. In this case, transmission to the human can be expected. In addition, there are some reports indicating that usage of vaccination in birds is a cause of mutation in the bird flu virus. The bird flu debate produces a number of uncertainties that science should help clear up. "How serious are chances that vaccinated poultry and other birds become silent carrier of bird flu?" and "Would this stand in the way of a vaccination policy?" are two questions that require a systematic approach to answer. In 2006, Savill et al. proposed a possible silent spread of H5N1 in vaccinated poultry [41]. Savill et al. reported that this silent spread could occur because of incomplete protection at the flock level, even if a vaccine was effective in individual birds [41]. They noted that the use of unvaccinated sentinels could mitigate, although not completely eliminate, the problem [41]. The spread of H5N1 and its likely reintroduction to domestic poultry increase the need for good agricultural vaccines [42]. Webster et al. said that the root cause of the continuing H5N1 pandemic threat might be the way the pathogenicity of H5N1 viruses is masked by co-circulating influenza viruses or bad agricultural vaccines [42]. One way to mitigate current concerns is to develop an influenza vaccine that is fully functional against drift influenza viruses [43].

Based on the basic principle of vaccination, a vaccine can generate immunity in those vaccinated by two main alternatives, via humoral or via cellular immunity mechanisms. Humoral immunity acts via antibody for clearance of viremia. The functional activity of serum antibody had been shown previously to reflect the state of resistance to influenza more accurately than antibody concentration [44]. Naikhin et al. noted that the quantitative parameters of the functional activity of antibody are directly related to the antigen dose and frequency of antigenic stimulation [44]. Cellular immunity act via lymphocyte and cytokine for clearance of infected cell. Swain et al. highlighted the multifaceted roles of CD4+ effector and memory T cells in protective responses to influenza infection and supported the concept that efficient priming of CD4+ T cells that react to shared influenza proteins could contribute greatly to vaccine strategies for influenza [45]. A good bird flu vaccine must have these two properties. However, and ideal vaccine has never been found.

Bird Flu Vaccination for Humans

In general, due to the burden of influenza hospitalizations among children, inactivated influenza vaccine is now routinely recommended for children age 6 to 59 months [46]. Live attenuated influenza vaccine is available for healthy persons 5 to 49 years of age. Although general human influenza vaccine is available there is no human bird flu vaccine [47]. Pandemics occur when influenza viruses undergo either antigenic drift or antigenic shift that results in a new viral strain that infects humans, when they are capable of sustained transmission from person-to-person, and when they are introduced in populations with little or no preexisting immunity. The influenza pandemic of 1918 caused an estimated 20-40 million deaths worldwide [48]. Vaccination is the best option by which spread of a pandemic virus could be prevented and severity of disease reduced. Production of live attenuated and inactivated vaccine seed viruses against avian influenza viruses, which have the potential to cause pandemics, and their testing in preclinical studies and clinical trials will establish the principles and ensure manufacturing experience that will be critical in the event of the emergence of such a virus into the human population [49]. To develop a H1N1 specific vaccine for humans is a new challenging topic in medicine at present. There is no success at present (2007). There is much ongoing research in this area.

In order to develop a new bird flu vaccine, advents in biotechnology can be applied [50]. Research into influenza vaccine covers main aspects including efficacy and safety. In addition to the classical immunological technique, with advent in bioinformatics, development of new influenza vaccine can be performed by advanced in silico techniques. Finding epitope is the first stage. To find a peptide candidate for a vaccine, the starting point is to find proper epitopes. Different procedures for epitope mapping are available at present [51]. It should be noted that synthetic peptide vaccines aiming at the induction of a protective response against malignant diseases are widely tested but despite their success in animal models they do not yet live up to their promise in humans [52]. Mapping for possible epitopes seems to be a hard step. The evidence accumulating from many recent studies points to a broader range of targets recognized than previously expected, in terms of both numbers and characteristics of the targeted antigens [53]. Also, multiple studies report a substantial variation in the targets recognized in different human individuals [53]. To solve the problem of heterogenicity, many new computational tools are developed for finding of possible candidate vaccine epitopes. Prediction of both T cell and B cell epitopes for further cancer vaccine development can be easily performed. Wiwanitkit recently predicted epitopes of

H5N1 bird flu virus by the bioinformatics method [54]. The result from this study can be useful information for further vaccine development. Development of new vaccine recombinant from alternative epitope is the next step. This can be done based on the principle of artificial genetic recombinant. To develop a new genetic recombinant, advanced gene delivery and transfer technique can be used. In addition to the classical artificial genetic recombinant generation, it can be performed by in silico mutating method. An in silico template for new vaccine recombinant can easily become available by simple mutation in sequence coding. Testing for new vaccine efficacy is the final step of vaccine development. Clinical trials should be performed before real generalization of the new vaccine. In order to decrease the long phase of clinical trial, the application of advanced medical informatics technology, gene ontology [55], can help predict the function or phenotypic expression of new developed vaccine. Schonbach et al. noted that support of vaccine development through textmining requires the timely development of domain-specific extraction rules for full-text articles, and a knowledge model for epitope-related information [56]. Johansson and Brett said that updating production capabilities with a shift in vaccination methods could allow for flexibility in the choice of antigen and decreased production time [57].

Bird Flu Chemoprophylaxis for Humans

Bird flu chemoprophylaxis for humans is indicated in health care workers who practiced with suspected animal and human infected cases [58]. A symposium organised by the Society of Infectious Disease (Singapore), Society of Intensive Care Medicine and the Singapore General Hospital was held in Singapore to gather the views of experts from Turkey, Thailand, Vietnam and Indonesia who collectively had first-hand experience in the management of the majority of cases of avian influenza worldwide [59]. The experts emphasized the importance of adapting international guidelines to the practicalities of situations on the ground [59]. There was stress on wide screening using clinical criteria primarily, molecular diagnostic techniques for diagnosis, and rational use of antiviral prophylaxis as well as infection control using at least surgical masks, gowns and gloves [59]. According to the World Health Organization, a strong recommendation to treat H5N1 patients with oseltamivir was made in part because of the severity of the disease and strong recommendations were also made to use neuraminidase inhibitors as chemoprophylaxis in high-risk exposure populations [58]. Lee et al. used a deterministic SEIR (susceptible-exposed-infectious-removed) meta-population model, together with scenario, sensitivity, and simulation analyses, to determine stockpiling strategies for neuraminidase inhibitors that would minimize absenteeism among healthcare workers [60]. They reported that earlier pandemic detection and initiation of prophylaxis might render shorter prophylaxis durations ineffective and eight weeks' prophylaxis substantially reduced peak absenteeism under a broad range of assumptions for severe pandemics (peak absenteeism > 10%) [60]. The effectiveness of oseltamivir and zanamivir for the therapy of clinical H5N1 influenza is questionable, simulation models suggest that a combination of targeted antiviral prophylaxis and quarantine might be able to contain an emerging influenza strain at the source [61]. Hayden and Pavia said that geographically targeted mass chemoprophylaxis might contain the spread of a pandemic virus, but multiple hurdles to successful implementation existed [62]. They noted that resistance to oseltamivir occurred with the H274Y variant in viruses that contain N1; however, such variants had been less fit, have not been transmitted from person to person, and had retained susceptibility to zanamivir [62]. They noted that alternative agents and approaches, including parenteral and combination therapy, for the treatment of influenza were needed in the near and long term [62]. To gauge the hazard presented by Tamiflu use during a pandemic, Singer et al. recommend a) direct measurement of Tamiflu persistence, biodegradation, and transformation in the environment, and b) further modeling of likely drug concentrations in the catchments of countries where humans and waterfowl come into frequent dose contact, and where significant Tamiflu deployment is envisaged [63].

Universal Precautions and Respiratory Precautions for Bird Flu

Universal precautions are a basic rule in medicine and can be used in the case of bird flu. In addition, since bird flu is a respiratory infection, respiratory precautions are also needed. Encourage the use of protective gear, such as gloves and masks, when treating patients with coughs or colds [64 - 65]. Have staffs that are ill stay at home, rather than risk exposure of colleagues and patients [64]. Key recommendations include admission to an isolation ward, cohorting of confirmed cases, hand hygiene with antiseptic solutions, use of N95 type masks, non-sterile disposable gloves and eye protection equipment during examination or when performing aerosols-generating procedures [66]. Use of patient-exclusive clinical instruments, daily disinfection of the hospital ward, implementation of measures to reduce risk of needle stick injuries and eye splashing, and reinforcement of appropriate sampling and transport of blood and other corporal fluids, are also recommended [66]. Skowronski et al. said that multiple back-up precautions, including oseltamivir prophylaxis, might prevent human infections and should be readily accessible and consistently used by those involved in the control of future outbreaks of avian influenza in poultry [67].

According to Guidelines for preventing health-care-associated pneumonia, 2003, the new recommendations include the addition of oseltamivir (to amantadine and rimantadine) for prophylaxis of all patients without influenza illness and oseltamivir and zanamivir (to amantadine and rimantadine) as treatment for patients who are acutely ill with influenza in a unit where an influenza outbreak is recognized [68]. Using a mask is an important protective behavior in the prevention of influenza. In theory, influenza viruses can be transmitted through aerosols, large droplets, or direct contact with secretions or fomites [69]. Published evidence indicates that aerosol transmission of influenza can be an important mode of transmission, which has obvious implications for pandemic influenza planning and in particular for recommendations about the use of N95 respirators as part of personal protective equipment [69]. Mardimae et al. reported that the N95 O2 mask, but not the nonrebreathing mask, provided the same efficiency of filtration of internal and external particles as the original N95, regardless of O2 flow into the mask [70]. Mardimae et al. also concluded that an N95 mask can be modified to administer a clinically equivalent FiO2 to a non-rebreathing mask while maintaining its filtration and isolation capabilities [70]. Li et al. reported that N95 respirators provided higher in-vivo filtration efficiency of 97% with significant reduction of air permeability and water vapor permeability [71]. They noted that the nano-masks could provide additional protective functions in stopping capillary diffusion and antibacterial activities compared to normal surgical masks/respirators [71]. Considering the nanostructure of N95, it can confirm the effectiveness in the prevention of viral particle transmission. [72].

Environmental Disinfection

Environmental disinfection is a widely used protocol for prevention of respiratory infection. There are many methods for environmental disinfection. The widely used methods include fumigation with formaldehyde, ozone application and ultraviolet (UV) application. The procedure of fumigation of a known contaminated area following spillage or handling of a biological agent is widely used in medicine [73]. This must include areas outside a laboratory such as hospital wards or ambulances that require fumigation [73]. However, there is no scientific proof that fumigation can or cannot result in the decontamination of the H5N1 virus. For UV application, Chumpolbanchorn et al. reported that UV light could not destroy the infectivity of the H5N1 virus even after exposure for 4 hours [74].

References

[1]   Sorrell EM, Ramirez-Nieto GC, Gomez-Osorio IG, Perez DR. Genesis of pandemic influenza. *Cytogenet. Genome Res.* 2007;117(1-4):394-402.

[2]   Thomas Y, Wunderli W, Cherpillod P, Kaiser L. Will avian influenza virus become a human virus? *Rev. Med. Suisse.* 2007 Apr 11;3(106):918-23.

[3]   Cox MM. Vaccines in development against avian influenza. *Minerva Med.* 2007 Apr;98(2):145-53.

[4]   Beck LH. Update in preventive medicine. *Ann Intern Med.* 2001 Jan 16;134(2):128-35.

[5]   Campbell S. Avian influenza: are you prepared? *Nurs. Stand.* 2006 Oct 11-17;21(5): 51-6.

[6]   Collignon PJ, Carnie JA. Infection control and pandemic influenza. *Med. J. Aust.* 2006 Nov 20;185(10 Suppl):S54-7.

[7]   Collins N, Litt J, Moore M, Winzenberg T, Shaw K. General practice: professional preparation for a pandemic. *Med. J. Aust.* 2006 Nov 20;185(10 Suppl):S66-9.

[8]   Capua I. Avian influenza--past, present and future challenges. *Dev. Biol.* (Basel). 2006;124:15-20.

[9]   Willis BC, Wortley P. Nurses' attitudes and beliefs about influenza and the influenza vaccine: a summary of focus groups in Alabama and Michigan. *Am. J. Infect. Control.* 2007 Feb;35(1):20-4.

[10]   Esposito S, Tremolati E, Bellasio M, Chiarelli G, Marchisio P, Tiso B, Mosca F, Pardi G, Principi N; V.I.P. Study Group. Attitudes and knowledge regarding influenza vaccination among hospital health workers caring for women and children. *Vaccine.* 2007 Jul 20;25(29):5283-9.

[11] Daley MF, Crane LA, Chandramouli V, Beaty BL, Barrow J, Allred N, Berman S, Kempe A. Misperceptions about influenza vaccination among parents of healthy young children. *Clin. Pediatr.* (Phila). 2007 Jun;46(5):408-17.

[12] Kristiansen IS, Halvorsen PA, Gyrd-Hansen D. Influenza pandemic: perception of risk and individual precautions in a general population. Cross sectional study. *BMC Public Health.* 2007 Apr 2;7:48.

[13] Al-Shehri AS, Abdel-Fattah M, Hifnawy T. Knowledge and concern about avian influenza among secondary school students in Taif, Saudi Arabia. *East Mediterr. Health J.* 2006;12 Suppl 2:S178-88.

[14] Al-Turki YA. Awareness of avian influenza ("bird flu") among attendees of a primary healthcare clinic in Riyadh. *Ann. Saudi Med.* 2006 May-Jun;26(3):245-7.

[15] Lau JT, Kim JH, Tsui HY, Griffiths S. Anticipated and current preventive behaviors in response to an anticipated human-to-human H5N1 epidemic in the Hong Kong Chinese general population. *BMC Infect. Dis.* 2007 Mar 15;7:18.

[16] Lau JT, Kim JH, Tsui H, Griffiths S. Perceptions related to human avian influenza and their associations with anticipated psychological and behavioral responses at the onset of outbreak in the Hong Kong Chinese general population. *Am. J. Infect. Control.* 2007 Feb;35(1):38-49.

[17] Fielding R, Lam WW, Ho EY, Lam TH, Hedley AJ, Leung GM. Avian influenza risk perception, Hong Kong. *Emerg. Infect. Dis.* 2005 May;11(5):677-82.

[18] Leggat PA, Mills D, Speare R. Hostellers' knowledge of transmission and prevention of avian influenza when travelling abroad. *Travel Med. Infect. Dis.* 2007 Jan;5(1):53-6.

[19] Abbate R, Di Giuseppe G, Marinelli P, Angelillo IF. Knowledge, attitudes, and practices of avian influenza, poultry workers, Italy. *Emerg. Infect. Dis.* 2006 Nov;12(11):1762-5.

[20] Capua I. Vaccination for notifiable avian influenza in poultry. *Rev. Sci. Tech.* 2007 Apr;26(1):217-27.

[21] Cox MM. Vaccines in development against avian influenza. *Minerva Med.* 2007 Apr;98(2):145-53.

[22] Capua I, Marangon S. Control of avian influenza in poultry. *Emerg. Infect. Dis.* 2006 Sep;12(9):1319-24.

[23] Horimoto T, Kawaoka Y. Strategies for developing vaccines against H5N1 influenza A viruses. *Trends Mol. Med.* 2006 Nov;12(11):506-14.

[24] Capua I, Marangon S. Control of avian influenza infections in poultry with emphasis on vaccination. *Expert Rev. Anti. Infect. Ther.* 2006 Oct;4(5):751-7.

[25] Capua I, Alexander DJ. The challenge of avian influenza to the veterinary community. *Avian Pathol.* 2006 Jun;35(3):189-205.

[26] Horimoto T, Kawaoka Y. Strategies for developing vaccines against H5N1 influenza A viruses. *Trends Mol. Med.* 2006 Nov;12(11):506-14.

[27] Swayne DE. Vaccines for List A poultry diseases: emphasis on avian influenza. *Dev. Biol.* (Basel). 2003;114:201-12.

[28] Bublot M, Pritchard N, Swayne DE, Selleck P, Karaca K, Suarez DL, Audonnet JC, Mickle TR. Development and use of fowlpox vectored vaccines for avian influenza. *Ann. N Y Acad. Sci.* 2006 Oct;1081:193-201.

[29] Bublot M, Pritchard N, Cruz JS, Mickle TR, Selleck P, Swayne DE. Efficacy of a fowlpox-vectored avian influenza H5 vaccine against Asian H5N1 highly pathogenic avian influenza virus challenge. *Avian Dis.* 2007 Mar;51(1 Suppl):498-500.

[30] Karaca K, Swayne DE, Grosenbaugh D, Bublot M, Robles A, Spackman E, Nordgren R. Immunogenicity of fowlpox virus expressing the avian influenza virus H5 gene (TROVAC AIV-H5) in cats. *Clin. Diagn. Lab. Immunol.* 2005 Nov;12(11):1340-2.

[31] Steensels M, Van Borm S, Lambrecht B, De Vriese J, Le Gros FX, Bublot M, van den Berg T. Efficacy of an inactivated and a fowlpox-vectored vaccine in Muscovy ducks against an Asian H5N1 highly pathogenic avian influenza viral challenge. *Avian Dis.* 2007 Mar;51(1 Suppl):325-31.

[32] Bublot M, Le Gros FX, Nieddu D, Pritchard N, Mickle TR, Swayne DE. Efficacy of two H5N9-inactivated vaccines against challenge with a recent H5N1 highly pathogenic avian influenza isolate from a chicken in Thailand. *Avian Dis.* 2007 Mar;51(1 Suppl):332-7.

[33] Laddy DJ, Yan J, Corbitt N, Kobasa D, Kobinger GP, Weiner DB. Immunogenicity of novel consensus-based DNA vaccines against avian influenza. *Vaccine.* 2007 Apr 20;25(16):2984-9.

[34] Lee CW, Senne DA, Suarez DL. Development and application of reference antisera against 15 hemagglutinin subtypes of influenza virus by DNA vaccination of chickens. *Clin. Vaccine Immunol.* 2006 Mar;13(3):395-402.

[35] Kodihalli S, Haynes JR, Robinson HL, Webster RG. Cross-protection among lethal H5N2 influenza viruses induced by DNA vaccine to the hemagglutinin. *J. Virol.* 1997 May;71(5):3391-6.

[36] Le Gall-Recule G, Cherbonnel M, Pelotte N, Blanchard P, Morin Y, Jestin V. Importance of a prime-boost DNA/protein vaccination to protect chickens against low-pathogenic H7 avian influenza infection. *Avian Dis.* 2007 Mar;51(1 Suppl):490-4.

[37] Sylte MJ, Hubby B, Suarez DL. Influenza neuraminidase antibodies provide partial protection for chickens against high pathogenic avian influenza infection. *Vaccine.* 2007 May 10;25(19):3763-72.

[38] Kodihalli S, Sivanandan V, Nagaraja KV, Shaw D, Halvorson DA. A type-specific avian influenza virus subunit vaccine for turkeys: induction of protective immunity to challenge infection. *Vaccine.* 1994 Nov;12(15):1467-72.

[39] Landman WJ, Schrier CC. Avian influenza: eradication from commercial poultry is still not in sight. *Tijdschr Diergeneeskd.* 2004 Dec 1;129(23):782-96.

[40] Ellis TM, Leung CY, Chow MK, Bissett LA, Wong W, Guan Y, Malik Peiris JS. Vaccination of chickens against H5N1 avian influenza in the face of an outbreak interrupts virus transmission. *Avian Pathol.* 2004 Aug;33(4):405-12.

[41] Savill NJ, St Rose SG, Keeling MJ, Woolhouse ME. Silent spread of H5N1 in vaccinated poultry. *Nature.* 2006 Aug 17;442(7104):757.

[42] Webster RG, Peiris M, Chen H, Guan Y. H5N1 outbreaks and enzootic influenza. *Emerg. Infect. Dis.* 2006 Jan;12(1):3-8.

[43] Hasegawa H, Ichinohe T, Tamura S, Kurata T. Development of a mucosal vaccine for influenza viruses: preparation for a potential influenza pandemic. *Expert Rev. Vaccines.* 2007 Apr;6(2):193-201.

[44] Naikhin AN, Artem'eva SA, Ermachenko TA, Vybornykh EN, Kustikova IuG, Doroshenko EV, Katorgina LG, Denisov GM, Kim TN. Antibody functional activity in immunization with influenza vaccines. *Vopr. Virusol.* 1993 Sep-Dec;38(5):204-7.

[45] Swain SL, Agrewala JN, Brown DM, Jelley-Gibbs DM, Golech S, Huston G, Jones SC, Kamperschroer C, Lee WH, McKinstry KK, Roman E, Strutt T, Weng NP. CD4+ T-cell memory: generation and multi-faceted roles for CD4+ T cells in protective immunity to influenza. *Immunol. Rev.* 2006 Jun;211:8-22.

[46] Zimmerman RK. Recent changes in influenza vaccination recommendations, 2007. *J. Fam. Pract.* 2007 Feb;56(2 Suppl Vaccines):S12-7, C1.

[47] Subbarao K, Luke C. H5N1 viruses and vaccines. *PLoS Pathog.* 2007 Mar;3(3):e40.

[48] Ford SM, Grabenstein JD. Pandemics, avian influenza A (H5N1), and a strategy for pharmacists. *Pharmacotherapy.* 2006 Mar;26(3):312-22.

[49] Luke CJ, Subbarao K. Vaccines for pandemic influenza. *Emerg. Infect. Dis.* 2006 Jan;12(1):66-72.

[50] Wiwanitkit V. Current research on drugs and vaccines for fighting bird flu. *Trans R. Soc. Trop. Med. Hyg.* 2007 Jul 24;

[51] Corradin G. Antigen processing and presentation. *Immunol Lett.* 1990 Aug;25(1-3):11-3.

[52] Bijker MS, Melief CJ, Offringa R, van der Burg SH. Design and development of synthetic peptide vaccines: past, present and future. *Expert Rev. Vaccines.* 2007 Aug;6(4):591-603.

[53] Sette A, Peters B. Immune epitope mapping in the post-genomic era: lessons for vaccine development. *Curr. Opin. Immunol.* 2007 Feb;19(1):106-10.

[54] Wiwanitkit V. Predicted epitopes of H5N1 bird flu virus by bioinformatics method: a clue for further vaccine development. *Chin. Med. J.* (Engl). 2006 Oct 20;119(20):1760.

[55] Thomas PD, Mi H, Lewis S. Ontology annotation: mapping genomic regions to biological function. *Curr. Opin. Chem. Biol.* 2007 Feb;11(1):4-11.

[56] Schonbach C, Nagashima T, Konagaya A. Textmining in support of knowledge discovery for vaccine development. *Methods.* 2004 Dec;34(4):488-95.

[57] Johansson BE, Brett IC. An inactivated subvirion influenza A (H5N1) vaccine. *N. Engl. J. Med.* 2006 Jun 22;354(25):2724-5

[58] Schunemann HJ, Hill SR, Kakad M, Bellamy R, Uyeki TM, Hayden FG, Yazdanpanah Y, Beigel J, Chotpitayasunondh T, Del Mar C, Farrar J, Tran TH, Ozbay B, Sugaya N, Fukuda K, Shindo N, Stockman L, Vist GE, Croisier A, Nagjdaliyev A, Roth C, Thomson G, Zucker H, Oxman AD; WHO Rapid Advice Guideline Panel on Avian Influenza.WHO Rapid Advice Guidelines for pharmacological management of sporadic human infection with avian influenza A (H5N1) virus. *Lancet Infect. Dis.* 2007 Jan;7(1):21-31.

[59] Lye DC, Nguyen DH, Giriputro S, Anekthananon T, Eraksoy H, Tambyah PA.Practical management of avian influenza in humans. *Singapore Med. J.* 2006 Jun;47(6):471-5.

[60] Lee VJ, Chen MI. Effectiveness of neuraminidase inhibitors for preventing staff absenteeism during pandemic influenza. *Emerg. Infect. Dis.* 2007 Mar;13(3):449-57.

[61] Gras-Masse H, Willand N. Neuraminidase inhibitors and risk of H5N1 influenza. *Ann Pharm Fr.* 2007 Jan;65(1):50-7.

[62] Hayden FG, Pavia AT. Antiviral management of seasonal and pandemic influenza. *J. Infect. Dis.* 2006 Nov 1;194 Suppl 2:S119-26.

[63] Singer AC, Nunn MA, Gould EA, Johnson AC. Potential risks associated with the proposed widespread use of Tamiflu. *Environ. Health Perspect.* 2007 Jan;115(1):102-6.

[64] Goldrick BA, Goetz AM. Pandemic influenza: what infection control professionals should know. *Am. J. Infect. Control.* 2007 Feb;35(1):7-13.

[65] Bird flu pandemic may not be certainty, but it's not too early to start preparing. *ED Manag.* 2005 Dec;17(12):133-6.

[66] Fica C A, Cifuentes D M, Ajenjo H MC, Delpiano M L, Febre V N, Medina L W, Parada E Y. Precautions in the care of patients hospitalized with H5N1 avian influenza. *Rev. Chilena Infectol.* 2006 Dec;23(4):290-6.

[67] Skowronski DM, Li Y, Tweed SA, Tam TW, Petric M, David ST, Marra F, Bastien N, Lee SW, Krajden M, Brunham RC. Protective measures and human antibody response during an avian influenza H7N3 outbreak in poultry in British Columbia, Canada. *CMAJ.* 2007 Jan 2;176(1):47-53.

[68] Tablan OC, Anderson LJ, Besser R, Bridges C, Hajjeh R; CDC; Healthcare Infection Control Practices Advisory Committee. Guidelines for preventing health-care--associated pneumonia, 2003: recommendations of CDC and the Healthcare Infection Control Practices Advisory Committee. *MMWR Recomm. Rep.* 2004 Mar 26;53(RR-3):1-36.

[69] Tellier R. Review of aerosol transmission of influenza A virus. *Emerg. Infect. Dis.* 2006 Nov;12(11):1657-62.

[70] Mardimae A, Slessarev M, Han J, Sasano H, Sasano N, Azami T, Fedorko L, Savage T, Fowler R, Fisher JA. Modified N95 mask delivers high inspired oxygen concentrations while effectively filtering aerosolized microparticles. *Ann. Emerg. Med.* 2006 Oct;48(4):391-9, 399.e1-2.

[71] Li Y, Wong T, Chung J, Guo YP, Hu JY, Guan YT, Yao L, Song QW, Newton E. In vivo protective performance of N95 respirator and surgical facemask. *Am. J. Ind. Med.* 2006 Dec;49(12):1056-65.

[72] Wiwanitkit V. N-95 face mask for prevention of bird flu virus: an appraisal of nanostructure and implication for infectious control. *Lung.* 2006 Nov-Dec;184(6):373-4.

[73] Tearle P. Decontamination by fumigation. *Commun. Dis. Public Health.* 2003 Jun;6(2):166-8.

[74] Chumpolbanchorn K, Suemanotham N, Siripara N, Puyati B, Chaichoune K. The effect of temperature and UV light on infectivity of avian influenza virus (H5N1, Thai field strain) in chicken fecal manure. *Southeast Asian J. Trop. Med. Public Health.* 2006 Jan;37(1):102-5.

Chapter 11

Effect of Emerging Bird Flu on the General Population

How were the Outbreaks Dealt With?

A. Medical and Public Health Response

Since there is a system of disease surveillance in all countries, many infectious diseases including botulism are on the list of the diseases under surveillance to be reported. Once the outbreak occurred, the patients were delivered to the local hospital and got the diagnosis. Usually, the presumptive diagnosis of botulism was based on clinical history and physical examination. Transfer to the tertiary hospital for proper management was performed in each outbreak. Final diagnosis was performed according to the results reported by the reference medical laboratory. The record and announcement of botulism as well as disease control was the next step. For disease control process, the practical protocols in medical epidemiology were usually followed. Identification of the source of outbreak, control of pathogen, treating of patients as well as prevention for further transmission was done.

B. Social Response to the Outbreak

Usually, the news of outbreaks was reported broadcast via several media including radio and television in the acute phase of outbreak. The avoidance of chicken and chicken product eating by the general population as a panic response to the news could be observed. Indeed, this pattern of response is a classical pattern of psychological response to any epidemic [1-2]. Many health education programs are broadcast to the local population at this phase. However, the continuation of this event is not observed and the social response when the time passes, is usually decreased. Concerning the political dimension, some clear directions in responding to the epidemic in medicine such as: 1) strong research and education campaigns; 2) close contact with political colleagues, interest groups and the community; 3) a national strategy which enjoins diverse interest groups, with courage, rationality and compassion, are also used [3]. Public information campaigns on television and the launching of several funding plans for research on bird flu in Thailand are good examples of those political responses to the most recent outbreak.

Bird Flu Panic [4 – 11]

Since 2004, bird flu has become a new infection with high fatality rates in humans living in Vietnam and Thailand. Most infected cases usually developed progressive pneumonia with acute respiratory distress syndrome and then consequently died. The main clinical manifestation of this infection is fever and flu-like symptoms. This disease has become an important disease under surveillance. It is recommended that any patients presenting with flu-like symptoms and with a history of direct avian contact should be further investigated by health care workers [12]. Repeated broadcasting of the virulence of atypical bird flu infection can result in some psychological effects on the general population. A common reaction is avoidance of eating avian products despite their being well cooked. Recently Wiwantkit reported a case of "bird flu panic", an example of a maladaptive psychological response to the rumors of bird flu in Thailand [13]. In this case of "bird flu panic," the diagnostic processes began with observation that there were no actual physical flu-like symptoms and also that the patient expressed excessive fear of bird flu infection [13]. In this case, if no careful history taking and physical examination were performed, a number of unnecessary laboratory investigations including complete blood count (CBC), serological test, viral culture, as well as PCR assays for H5N1 could be expected [13]. Indeed, bird flu infection is a viral infection and the disease occurs rarely after a week of contact [13]. In addition, only living or visiting in the area of outbreak without a history of close contact with infected chickens has never been reported to be a mode of transmission of bird flu [13]. Without of course, minimizing the potential severity of actual bird flu, clinicians should consider that psychological symptoms can occur during times of bird flu outbreak that are not due to physical symptoms from bird flu and may just be a psychological reaction to the presence of bird flu [13].

If an influenza pandemic struck today, borders might close, the global economy would be severely impacted, international vaccine supplies and health care systems would be overwhelmed, and some people might panic [14]. According to Guangdong provincial seminar on avian influenza and influenza, the specialists concluded that the media should report the news objectively and issue the public warnings against avian influenza after consulting specialists, so as to avoid unnecessary social panic [15]. The Royal Academy for Medicine of Belgium said that the effectiveness of antiviral treatment and prophylaxis during a pandemic was, given the lack of experience, uncertain [16]. The Royal Academy for Medicine of Belgium noted that the fact that such remedies would be available should not create a false sense of security and should certainly not lead to reduced alertness with regard to the preparation and implementation of other measures, and panic reactions among the population should be avoided [16]. Lau et al. concluded that panic and interruption of daily routines might occur in the event of a human avian influenza outbreak [17]. Lau et al. noted that dissemination of accurate, timely information would reduce unnecessary distress and unwanted behaviors [17]. Ensuring for no panic is an important part of infection control [18].

Change of Folkway in Management of in-House Avian Farming [19 - 23]

In-home farming is a widely distributed farming system in Southeast Asia where the recent H5N1 influenza epidemic occurred. The effect of the recent epidemic on the chicken farm can be divided into many phases. In the accent epiclesis phase, the chickens at the farms were killed. Millions of chickens were destroyed. A sudden decrease in the amount of the total chicken population in Southeast Asian countries could be demonstrated. This causes the ban erupting on many chicken farms. The owners of in-house chicken farms seem to be greatly effected due to the disease-control protocol, especially in the killing of suspected animals around epidemic sites. These practices cause the in-house farms' owners in epidemic areas to lose all of their chickens. Since these farmers are usually in the low socioeconomic status population, they are too poor to buy new chickens for feeding in their farms and this shifts the burden to the local governments. In Thailand the local government has to pay millions for the farmers who lost their chicken due to disease control protocol. On the other hand, there were some areas without epidemic. In these areas, the farmers still have their healthy chickens. But they faced many problems in trying to sell their chickens and chicken products. The limitation on avian transportation by the government board obstructed the transferring. In some areas where transportation is possible, the wide rumors among the local population made them avoid ingestion of chicken. These factors also affected the incomes of the owners of in-house farming in non epidemic areas.

There are two main groups of in-house avian farms in Southeast Asia - chicken farms and duck farms. The in-house chicken farm is usually set on the grounds surrounding the houses. Back yard chicken is a basic source of food for the local farmer. A poor vaccination system is usually applied. The recent epidemic mainly hit the back yard chickens. Since the back yard chicken usually live near the house and can have contact with local villagers and with animals in homes, the control of the in-house farming scepter is needed. Many protocols were set to increase knowledge of local villagers about in-house farming directives for recent epidemics. Some villagers adapted their behavior in farming while the others abandoned in-house farming. Another interesting point in in-house chicken farming is fighting-cock farming [24]. This is a local sport in Thailand. The price of fighting cocks is a hundred times more than back yard chickens. These cocks have to be moved to a distance local stadium for fighting. If those cocks were silent carriers of H5N1 influenza, the spread of disease can be expected. Summative, fighting cocks' owners have close contact with their cocks. They usually kiss and usually suck mucous from the noses of the fighting cocks. This group of chickens is very hard to control. Due to high prices, the owners of fighting cocks usually act against the infection control process of the local government. Responding to the recent epidemic, a specific protocol for this population of chicken was set in Thailand. Disease surveillance system and chicken identification cards were proposed for control of transportation of fighting cocks to fight in a distant fighting stadium.

Concerning in-house farming for ducks, in-house duck farms are usually located in the rice field and swamp around the local village. This fact means the in-house duck farm is a high risk for H5N1 influenza virus contact. Spreading of the virus into the environment is easy if there is an epidemic among these ducks. In the recent epidemic in Thailand, millions of these ducks were killed. Similar situation as in-house back yard chicken farms in the recent epidemic control could be demonstrated. An interesting point on in-house duck farming is that although there were epidemics and the local government gave several education sessions on a good farming system, local villages still persist in their old habit of folkway of leaving their ducks in the rice fields. Concerning the chronic effect of H5N1 epidemics, many affected countries had to face up to a considerable loss in the farming economy. Banning of avian products from other countries hit the structure of the farming economy in affected countries. Several medium and large chicken farms closed. For the general population, a rooted fear of chicken ingestion persisted in their mind for years. Of interest, the local in-house farming system recovered to be a folkway in distant rural villages.

Impact on Tourism

After broadcasting news on H5N1 epidemics, a sudden impact on tourism in affected countries occurred. Tourist programs were cancelled. A precautionary rule was set for many countries. Similar to the epidemic of SARS, there are protocols for surveillance of a suspected person form affected countries in the immigration process. Within the affected countries, the local people feared for traveling to epidemic areas, and this actively hinted the economy of epidemic areas. Some tourist attractions in non epidemic areas got no visits from tourists. These places include natural bird parks and zoos. In Thailand, after the episode of tiger H5N1 infection near Pattaya, no tourist visited the zoo. Many zoos had to close for a while in order to closely observe the animals and to prevent H5N1 contamination from outside. Concerning natural bird parks, some were closed and followed an infection control process. This brought a great loss of natural treasures. Since many natural bird parks contain migrant birds from distant areas and can be the sources of the H5N1 virus, several protocols were set for further control and surveillance of these lands. However, the proper method balancing between natural treasure protection and disease control is still in being sought.

Indeed, the outbreaks of influenza among tourists have been documented for a long time. Uyeki et al. investigated a large summertime outbreak of acute respiratory illness during May-September 1998 in Alaska and the Yukon Territory, Canada [25]. Uyeki et al. noted that modern travel patterns might facilitate similar outbreaks, indicating the need for increased awareness about influenza by health care providers and travelers, and the desirability of year-round influenza surveillance in some regions [25]. Perz et al. reported a pre-seasonal outbreak of influenza-like illness in a tourist group that had returned from Ireland to the United States on October 1 and 2, 1999 [26]. Perz et al. concluded that international travelers, particularly older persons and members of organized tour groups, might experience increased risks for respiratory viral infection [26]. Perz et al. noted that the recognition and containment of imported infectious diseases depend on prompt reporting and epidemiologic investigation [26]. On June 18, 1999, CDC and Health Canada received reports from public health authorities in Alaska and the Yukon Territory about clusters of febrile respiratory illness and associated pneumonia among travelers and tourism workers [27]. Another influenza B virus outbreak on a cruise ship in Northern Europe (2000) was also reported by CDC [28]. These reports also document the importance of influenza outbreak in travelers [27 - 28].

In travel medicine, influenza is a big concern [29]. Dick et al. said that one third of persons who traveled abroad experienced a travel-related illness, usually diarrhea or an upper respiratory infection [30]. Medical advice for patients planning trips abroad must be individualized and based on the most current expert recommendations [30]. It is increasingly clear that travelers, while at risk for infections, also play a role in the global dispersal of pathogens [31]. According to the recommendations of the National Action Committee on Immunization and the Committee to Advise on Tropical Medicine and Travel in Canada Communicable Disease Reports, the Canadian Immunization Guide, Laboratory Centre for Disease Control, United States Centres for Disease Control, and World Health Organization, the elderly should be vaccinated against influenza [32 - 36]. An increasing number of individuals undertake air travel annually [37 - 39]. Leder and Newman said that issues regarding cabin air quality and the potential risks of transmission of respiratory infections during flight had been investigated and debated previously, but, with the advent of severe acute respiratory syndrome and influenza outbreaks, these issues had recently taken on heightened importance [37]. Hogg and Huston said that because the outbreak of an influenza pandemic was likely imminent, implementing standard guidelines for control of respiratory infections in primary care offices seemed reasonable [40]. They noted that following these guidelines would help prevent patients and staff from contracting serious respiratory illnesses [40]. Heudrof et al. noted that public health authorities should improve and increase their publicity campaigns for travel health and vaccination in order to prevent travel-associated influenza [41].

Recently, Legatt et al. reported that hostellers attending the travelers' information night in Australia reported having moderate concern about avian influenza and those hostellers also had a variable knowledge of the sources of infection of avian influenza [42]. Leggat et al. said that although hostellers responded positively to hand washing advice provided in the travel health lecture, reinforcement of other possible measures to prevent avian influenza, particularly the possible role of antiviral drugs, might be needed [42]. Legatt et al. noted that accurate and relevant information in an acceptable format could play an important role in supporting this group [43]. Leggat et al. concluded that it was important that policies being promoted by travel health advocacy groups continue to advocate that travelers seeked travel health advice from a qualified source early, preferably around 6 to 8 weeks before travel, and that personal safety be discussed as part of the travel health consultation [43].

Economic Impact of Bird Flu

As previously mentioned, the economic impact of influenza is well documented [44 - 52]. Controlling outbreaks in domestic fowl and limiting contact between humans and infected birds must be the priorities in the management of this disease at the public health level [53]. The killing of suspected poultry costs a lot as previously mentioned [54]. Clague et al. conducted a province-wide household survey using two-stage cluster sampling to determine the burden of influenza-like illness in Sa Kaeo Province, Thailand [55]. Clague et al. used the total number of reported influenza that occurred in May 2003 and a prospective study of outpatient influenza in clinic patients to develop an estimate of the annualized incidence of influenza [55]. According to this work, the total individual cost per illness episode was 663 baht (15.78 US dollars) [55]. Akasawa performed similar research and reported that the average number of workdays missed due to influenza-like illness was 1.30 days, and the average work loss was valued at 137 US dollars per person [56]. This is a considerable loss. Carrat et al. confirmed the substantial burden of illness of influenza [57]. These results on loss due to infection should be useful for evaluating the cost-effectiveness of strategies against influenza. Fasina et al. said that control of highly pathogenic avian influenza H5N1 would best be understood by policy makers in financial terms [58]. Fasia et al. concluded that effective control through vaccination of poultry was much cheaper and reduced the chances of human illness, and poultry vaccination combined with other control measures would be the most effective means of control in most developing economies [58].

Political Impact of Bird Flu

Political impact of bird flu should also be a concern. Political fiction in dealing with a bird flu epidemic could be seen [59]. Kunze et al. noted that a sudden influenza pandemic would give rise to a number of grave problems in the medical field (increase in mortality rates) as well as in social and political areas (maintaining the infrastructure of the country) [60]. In light of this fact it appears necessary to investigate the possibility of an influenza pandemic and to take suitable precautionary measures [60]. Risk assessment estimates the probability of a pandemic, the options available for control, and the relative benefits of those options as situations change [61]. Risk management is the political response to that assessment [61]. An important preventive measure for bird flu, vaccination, is widely discussed on the political aspect. In the event of a bioterrorist event or a pandemic flu outbreak, it might be necessary to ration vaccine or other treatments [62]. Fedson said that planning for pandemic vaccination should begin during the interpandemic period to ensure a vaccine supply that would be adequate to meet demand in all countries [63]. Fedson mentioned that this would require the skills not only of experts in virology, epidemiology and public health but also those in politics, economics and law [63 - 64]. The circumstances that contributed to the national and local vaccine shortage; the improvisation by health policymakers, hospital administrators, physicians, and nurses to prevent influenza cases despite the shortfall; and some of the legal, fiscal, logistical, social, and political pressures that local health professionals faced in deciding who should receive the limited supply of influenza vaccine are the areas to be investigated [62]. From the frontline of disease control their concerns about distribution of medicines and the inadequate stocks of anti-virals and vaccines must be taken into account [65]. Without this necessary buy-in doctors may find it difficult to balance their Hippocratic oath to treat all equally with the political necessity of treatment prioritization [65]. Kotalik said that examination of the pandemic plans of Canada, the UK and the USA, from an ethical perspective, raises several concerns [66]. Kotalik noted that scarcity of human and material resources was assumed to be severe and plans focused on prioritization but did not identify resources that would be optimally required to reduce deaths and other serious consequences, hence, these plans did not facilitate a truly informed choice at the political level where decisions had to be made on how much to invest now in order to reduce scarcity in case a pandemic occurred [66].

Bioterrorism by Bird Flu Virus: A New Concern

Epidemic and pandemic influenza is a new concern [67 - 80]. Krug et al. said that recent events highlighted the potential of influenza A virus as a bioterrorist weapon: the high virulence of the influenza A virus that infected people in Hong Kong in 1997; and the development of laboratory methods to generate influenza A viruses by transfection of DNAs without a helper virus [81]. Duley noted that the "all-hazards" planning currently being undertaken by the key health care system partners in Connecticut as a result of federal funding for preparedness, post 9/11, had fostered great working relationships between these entities and their local, regional, and statewide planning counterparts [82]. Duley said that many of the specific grant dollars being provided to these facilities could help set a plan needed to deal with pandemic bird flu [82]. Mair et al. said that the burden of annual influenza epidemics and the fragility and instability of the capacity to respond to them underscored the USA's ongoing vulnerability to pandemic influenza and highlighted gaps in bioterrorism preparedness and response efforts [83].

References

[1]   Boulougouris JC, Rabavilas AD, Stefanis CN, Vaidakis N, Tabouratzis DG. Epidemic faintness: a psychophysiological investigation. *Psychiatr. Clin.* (Basel). 1981;14(4):215-25.

[2]   Maunder R, Hunter J, Vincent L, Bennett J, Peladeau N, Leszcz M, Sadavoy J, Verhaeghe LM, Steinberg R, Mazzulli T. The immediate psychological and occupational impact of the 2003 SARS outbreak in a teaching hospital. *CMAJ.* 2003;168:1245-5.

[3]   Blewett N. Political dimensions of AIDS. *AIDS.* 1988;2 Suppl 1:S235-8.

[4]   Moscioni S. Stricken by panic or bird seed? *Recenti. Prog Med.* 2005 Nov;96(11):559.

[5]   Basu P. Panic over bird flu pandemic premature, experts say. *Nat. Med.* 2006 Mar;12(3):258.

[6]   Bonneux L, Van Damme W. An iatrogenic pandemic of panic. *BMJ.* 2006 Apr 1;332(7544):786-8.

[7]   Bird flu: don't fly into a panic. Whether the H5N1 virus will "make the jump" and spread among humans is uncertain, but here are some tips to protect yourself. *Harv. Health Lett.* 2006 Jun;31(8):1-3.

[8]   Richards G. Avian influenza: preparation not panic. *Prim. Care Respir. J.* 2006 Aug;15(4):217-8.

[9]   Nau JY. Washington's state of panic: 200 million dollars. *Rev. Med. Suisse.* 2006 Dec 6;2(90):2825.

[10] Kmietowicz Z. Political lead essential to avoid panic when flu strikes. *BMJ*. 2005 Nov 12;331(7525):1099.

[11] Manderscheid RW. reparing for pandemic Avian influenza: ensuring mental health services and mitigating panic. *Arch. Psychiatr. Nurs*. 2007 Feb;21(1):64-7.

[12] Chotpitayasunondh T, Lochindarat S, Srisan P. Preliminary clinical description of influenza A (H5N1) in Thailand. *W. Epidemiol. Surveil. Rep*. 2004; 35: 89-92.

[13] Wiwanitkit V. Bird flu panic: a case report. *Int. J. Mental Health*. 2007; 3 (2): 1.

[14] Pascoe N. A pandemic flu: not if, but when. SARS was the wake-up call we slept through. *Tex. Nurs*. 2006 Jan;80(1):6-10.

[15] Yu SY, Chen Q, Hu GF. Summary of Guangdong provincial seminar on avian influenza and influenza. *Di Yi Jun Yi Da Xue Xue Bao*. 2005 Dec;25(12):1587-8.

[16] Recommendation of the Royal Academy for Medicine of Belgium to the responsible policy authorities in connection with the continually increasing threat of an outbreak of an influenza epidemic. *Verh. K Acad. Geneeskd. Belg*. 2006;68(2):139-50.

[17] Lau JT, Kim JH, Tsui H, Griffiths S. Perceptions related to human avian influenza and their associations with anticipated psychological and behavioral responses at the onset of outbreak in the Hong Kong Chinese general population. *Am. J. Infect. Control*. 2007 Feb;35(1):38-49.

[18] How to develop and implement pandemic preparedness plans? The need for a coherent European policy. *Vaccine*. 2006 Nov 10;24(44-46):6766-9.

[19] Kaasschieter GA, de Jong R, Schiere JB, Zwart D. Towards a sustainable livestock production in developing countries and the importance of animal health strategy therein. *Vet Q*. 1992 Apr;14(2):66-75.

[20] Blackshaw JK. Objective measures of welfare in farming environments. *Aust. Vet. J*. 1986 Nov;63(11):361-4.

[21] Razumov SA, Gal'pern IL, Korovin KF. Cock fighting as a model of emotional stress. *Fiziol Zh SSSR Im I M Sechenova*. 1978 Oct;64(10):1372-81.

[22] Larkin M. Avian flu: sites seek to respond and reassure. *Lancet Infect. Dis*. 2005 Mar;5(3):141-2.

[23] Stone R. Avian influenza. Combating the bird flu menace, down on the farm. *Science*. 2006 Feb 17;311(5763):944-6.

[24] Yaowares Y. Cockfighting : the culture that has to change to avoid a deadly influenza pandemic. *Thai J. Acad. Pub. Heath*. 2006 May - Jun; 15 (3): 357-366.

[25] Uyeki TM, Zane SB, Bodnar UR, Fielding KL, Buxton JA, Miller JM, Beller M, Butler JC, Fukuda K, Maloney SA, Cetron MS; Alaska/Yukon Territory Respiratory Outbreak Investigation Team. Large summertime influenza A outbreak among tourists in Alaska and the Yukon Territory. *Clin Infect. Dis*. 2003 May 1;36(9):1095-102.

[26] Perz JF, Craig AS, Schaffner W. Mixed outbreak of parainfluenza type 1 and influenza B associated with tourism and air travel. *Int. J. Infect. Dis*. 2001;5(4):189-91.

[27] Centers for Disease Control and Prevention (CDC). Outbreak of influenza A infection among travelers--Alaska and the Yukon Territory, May-June 1999. *MMWR Morb. Mortal. Wkly Rep*. 1999 Jul 2;48(25):545-6, 555.

[28] Centers for Disease Control and Prevention (CDC). Influenza B virus outbreak on a cruise ship--Northern Europe, 2000. *MMWR Morb. Mortal. Wkly Rep.* 2001 Mar 2;50(8):137-40.

[29] The Committee to Advise on Tropical Medicine and Travel (CATMAT) and the National Advisory Committee on Immunization (NACI). Travel, influenza, and prevention. *Can. Commun. Dis. Rep.* 1996 Sep 1;22(17):141-5.

[30] Dick L. Travel medicine: helping patients prepare for trips abroad. *Am. Fam. Physician.* 1998 Aug;58(2):383-98, 401-2.

[31] Chen LH, Wilson ME. Recent Advances and New Challenges in Travel Medicine. *Curr. Infect. Dis. Rep.* 2002 Feb;4(1):50-58.

[32] Thomas RE. Preparing patients to travel abroad safely. Part 2: Updating vaccinations. *Can. Fam. Physician.* 2000 Mar;46:646-52, 655-6.

[33] Eickhoff TC. Adult immunizations: how are we doing? *Hosp. Pract.* (Minneap). 1996 Nov 15;31(11):107-8, 111-2, 115-7.

[34] Lauer DJ. Symposium on immunization. Problems of immunizing adults in foreign travel and in industry. *Arch. Environ. Health.* 1967 Oct;15(4):508-11.

[35] Beytout J, Laurichesse H. Adult immunization in France: an update. *Rev. Prat.* 2004 Mar 15;54(5):499-505.

[36] Lashley FR. Emerging infectious diseases: vulnerabilities, contributing factors and approaches. *Expert Rev. Anti. Infect. Ther.* 2004 Apr;2(2):299-316.

[37] Leder K, Newman D. Respiratory infections during air travel. *Intern. Med. J.* 2005 Jan;35(1):50-5.

[38] Factsheet. Avian influenza ('bird flu'). *N S W Public Health Bull.* 2006 Jul-Aug;17(7-8):121.

[39] Juckett G. Travel medicirne 2005. *W V. Med. J.* 2004 Nov-Dec;100(6):222-5.

[40] Hogg W, Huston P. Controlling droplet-transmitted respiratory infections: best practices and cost. *Can. Fam. Physician.* 2006 Oct;52(10):1229-32.

[41] Heudorf U, Tiarks-Jungk P, Stark S. Travel medicine and vaccination as a task of infection prevention--data of the special consultation hours of the public health department Frankfurt on the Main, Germany, 2002-2004. *Gesundheitswesen.* 2006 May;68(5):316-22.

[42] Leggat PA, Mills D, Speare R. Hostellers' knowledge of transmission and prevention of avian influenza when travelling abroad. *Travel Med. Infect. Dis.* 2007 Jan;5(1):53-6.

[43] Leggat PA, Mills D, Speare R. Level of concern and sources of information of a group of Brisbane hostelers for personal safety and terrorism when traveling abroad. *J. Travel Med.* 2007 Mar-Apr;14(2):112-6.

[44] Roden AT. Influenza as a national problem. *Postgrad. Med. J.* 1963 Oct;39:612-8.

[45] Korlof B. Economic aspects of the 1957-58 influenza epidemic in Sweden. Sven Lakartidn. 1959 Jul 3;56(27):1911-2

[46] Insurance claims and influenza. *Lancet.* 1953 Apr 11;1(15):735

[47] Public health; prescribed diseases; influenza; infectious disease in England and Wales. *Lancet.* 1951 Mar 10;1(10):593.

[48] Pestel M. Socioeconomic incidence of influenza. *Presse Med.* 1971 Oct 23;79(44):1994-5.

[49] Lamarca V. Socio-economic aspects of influenza and its prevention. *Folia Med.* (Napoli). 1972 Jun-Jul;54(6):120-8.

[50] Death claim payments more than 991,000,000 dollars in 1970. *Stat. Bull. Metropol. Life Insur. Co.* 1971 Mar;52:9-11.

[51] Patterson GD. The economics of illness. An employee sickness study. *Med. J. Aust.* 1969 Aug 2;2(5):249-52.

[52] Townson P. Cutting the cost of influenza. *Occup. Health* (Lond). 1970 Sep;22(9):299-302.

[53] Laranjeira CA. Avian influenza--a new challenge. *Bratisl. Lek. Listy.* 2006;107(11-12):412-7.

[54] Kanamori S, Jimba M. Compensation for avian influenza cleanup. *Emerg. Infect. Dis.* 2007 Feb;13(2):341-2.

[55] Clague B, Chamany S, Burapat C, Wannachaiwong Y, Simmerman JM, Dowell SF, Olsen SJ. A household survey to assess the burden of influenza in rural Thailand. *Southeast Asian J. Trop. Med. Public Health.* 2006 May;37(3):488-93.

[56] Akazawa M, Sindelar JL, Paltiel AD. Economic costs of influenza-related work absenteeism. *Value Health.* 2003 Mar-Apr;6(2):107-15.

[57] Carrat F, Sahler C, Rogez S, Leruez-Ville M, Freymuth F, Le Gales C, Bungener M, Housset B, Nicolas M, Rouzioux C. Influenza burden of illness: estimates from a national prospective survey of household contacts in France. *Arch. Intern. Med.* 2002 Sep 9;162(16):1842-8.

[58] Fasina FO, Meseko AC, Joannis TM, Shittu AI, Ularamu HG, Egbuji NA, Sulaiman LK, Onyekonwu NO. Control versus no control: options for avian influenza H5N1 in Nigeria. *Zoonoses Public Health.* 2007;54(5):173-6.

[59] Dubois G. Political fiction or a future scenario for a pandemic of influenza? *Eur. J. Epidemiol.* 1994 Aug;10(4):523.

[60] Kunze U, Dorner D, Groman E, Hartl H. Influenza pandemic: does Austria need an emergency plan? *Wien Med Wochenschr.* 1999;149(13):388-91.

[61] Dowdle WR. Pandemic influenza: confronting a re-emergent threat. The 1976 experience. *J. Infect. Dis.* 1997 Aug;176 Suppl 1:S69-72.

[62] Schoch-Spana M, Fitzgerald J, Kramer BR; UPMC Influenza Task Force. Influenza vaccine scarcity 2004-05: implications for biosecurity and public health preparedness. *Biosecur. Bioterror.* 2005;3(3):224-34.

[63] Fedson DS. Vaccination for pandemic influenza: a six point agenda for interpandemic years. *Pediatr. Infect. Dis. J.* 2004 Jan;23(1 Suppl):S74-7.

[64] Fedson DS. Pandemic influenza and the global vaccine supply. *Clin. Infect. Dis.* 2003 Jun 15;36(12):1552-61.

[65] Recommendations and guidelines on influenza vaccination and treatment. A key success factor. *Vaccine.* 2006 Nov 10;24(44-46):6783-4.

[66] Kotalik J. Preparing for an influenza pandemic: ethical issues. *Bioethics.* 2005 Aug;19(4):422-31.

[67] Epidemic and pandemic influenza, who cares and how? *Vaccine.* 2006 Nov 10;24(44-46):6762-5.

[68] Alibek K, Liu G. Biodefense shield and avian influenza. *Emerg. Infect. Dis.* 2006 May;12(5):873-5.

[69] Bernice JA. Bird flu: a real threat or media hype? *Clin. Leadersh. Manag. Rev.* 2006 Jul 25;20(4):E8.

[70] Jackson BA, Buehler JW, Cole D, Cookson S, Dausey DJ, Honess-Morreale L, Lance S, Molander RC, O'Neal P, Lurie N. Bioterrorism with zoonotic disease: public health preparedness lessons from a multiagency exercise. *Biosecur Bioterror.* 2006;4(3):287-92.

[71] Tseng SS. SARS, avian flu, bioterror: infection control awareness for the optometrist. *Clin. Exp. Optom.* 2007 Jan;90(1):31-5.

[72] Check E. Heightened security after flu scare sparks biosafety debate. *Nature.* 2005 Apr 21;434(7036):943.

[73] Mack TM. The ghost of pandemics past. *Lancet.* 2005 Apr 16-22;365(9468):1370-2.

[74] Phillips FB, Williamson JP. Local health department applies incident management system for successful mass influenza clinics. *J. Public Health Manag. Pract.* 2005 Jul-Aug;11(4):269-73.

[75] Ursano RJ. Preparedness for SARS, influenza, and bioterrorism. *Psychiatr. Serv.* 2005 Jan;56(1):7.

[76] Norrby SR. Alert to a European epidemic. *Nature.* 2004 Sep 30;431(7008):507-8.

[77] Alexander DA. Bioterrorism: preparing for the unthinkable. *J. R. Army Med. Corps.* 2003 Jun;149(2):125-30.

[78] Madjid M, Lillibridge S, Mirhaji P, Casscells W. Influenza as a bioweapon. *J. R. Soc. Med.* 2003 Jul;96(7):345-6

[79] There are two sides to biodefence. *Nature.* 2003 Apr 10;422(6932):545.

[80] Baxter RJ, Steinberg CR, Shapiro JR. Is the U.S. public health system ready for bioterrorism? An assessment of the U.S. public health infrastructure and its capacity for infectious disease surveillance. *Yale J. Health Policy Law Ethics.* 2001 Autumn; 2(1):1-21.

[81] Krug RM. The potential use of influenza virus as an agent for bioterrorism. *Antiviral Res.* 2003 Jan;57(1-2):147-50.

[82] Duley MG. The next pandemic: anticipating an overwhelmed health care system. *Yale J. Biol. Med.* 2005 Oct;78(5):355-62.

[83] Mair M, Grow RW, Mair JS, Radonovich LJ Jr. Universal influenza vaccination: the time to act is now. *Biosecur Bioterror.* 2006;4(1):20-40.

Chapter 12

Other Bird-Borne Infectious Diseases

What Is "Bird-Borne Infectious Disease?" [1 – 2]

A bird-borne infectious disease is defined as a disease that can be transmitted by birds. Birds might be the reservoir host or infection source. Humans might get the infection from direct or indirect contact with birds or their products. An important concern about bird-borne infections is that birds can fly for a long distance and some can migrate to new locations. Traveling of the birds can be the cause of new emerging infectious disease in the new retting. In addition, people have a custom of visiting lands, which might be the next source of infection, and the behavior can be the source of a new bird-borne disease epidemic. Several bacterial, viral, fungal, and parasitic organisms are mentioned as potential bird-borne zoonoses [2]. Salmonellosis, toxoplasmosis, and allergic alveolitis are also considered [2]. In addition to H5N1 avian influenza infection and other types of bird flu, there are also other bird-borne infections. Those important bird-borne infectious diseases will be hereby summarized and presented.

Cryptococcosis [3 - 12]

Cryptococcosis is a well-known fungal infection. The etiological agent of cryptococcosis is *Cryptococcus neofornans*. The etiologic agent is an encapsulated fungus. Naturally the *Cryptococcus neofornans* can be seen as a contaminant in bird feces. Despite recent advances in the genetics and molecular biology of C. neoformans, and improved techniques for molecular epidemiology, aspects of the ecology, population structure, and mode of reproduction of this environmental pathogen remain to be established [13]. *Cryptococcus neofornans* is a basidiomycetous fungus with a defined sexual cycle that has been linked to differentiation and virulence [14]. An ongoing genome sequencing project promises to reveal much about the evolution of this human fungal pathogen into three distinct varieties or species [14]. Hull and Heitman noted that *Cryptococcus neofornans* shares features with both model ascomycetous yeasts (*Saccharomyces cerevisiae*, *Schizosaccharomyces pombe*) and basidiomycetous pathogens and mushrooms (*Ustilago maydis*, *Coprinus cinereus*, *Schizophyllum commune*), yet ongoing studies reveal unique features associated with virulence and the arrangement of the mating type locus [14]. The epidemiology of cryptococcosis can primarily be explained by exposure to an infective aerosolized inoculum, such as basidiospores released from specific host plants and/or desiccated blastoconidia (yeast cells) disseminated from accumulations of dried pigeon dung [15 - 16]. As mentioned, the problematic bird species are pigeons and doves because these two kinds of birds are widely raised as domestic animals. Soogarun et al. recently studied the contamination within birds' excreta and reported that a high number of Cryptoccescal species contamination could be detected. According to this study [17], *Cryptococcus neoformans* var neoformans was recovered from pigeon excreta in 9.09% [17]. This implies those having impaired immunity may get this fungus from the environment [17]. A similar study was performed by Kielstein et al. [18]. According to this work, in 50% of the samples of pigeon excreta examined in Innsbruck (Austria), *Cryptococcus albidus* could be isolated but not *Cryptococcus neoformans* [18]. Kohno reported the isolated *Cryptococcus neofornans* from chicken feces in as many as at 70 % of the villages tested in his research [19]. Kohna noted that chicken as well as pigeon feces were believed to be an origin of infection [19].

After direct contact, *Cryptococcus neofornans* can act as a pathogen in an immununocompromised host [20 - 21]. Regarding cell-mediated immunity, CD4+ T cells are crucial for successful resistance, but CD8+ T cells may also participate significantly in the cytokine-mediated activation of anticryptococcal effector cells [22]. In addition to cell-mediated immunity, monoclonal antibodies to the major capsular polysaccharide, the glucuronoxylomannan, offer some protection in murine models of cryptococcosis [22]. Hence, impact of immune defect can lead to high vulnerability to cryptococcal infection. In the area of human's immunodeficiency virus (HIV) infection, Cryptococcus becomes an important opportunistic infection of HIV-infected patients [23 - 26]. Although cryptococcosis can manifest in several forms the most common form in HIV-infected patients is neurological manifestation [27 – 30]. The neurological infection due to *Cryptococcus neofornans* is a chronic infection process. The headache is a common complaint. Positive meningeal signs can be detected in the infected population. The definitive diagnosis can be performed by microscopic examination of cerebrospinal fluid (CSF) [31 – 32]. Concerning the CSF in the infected case, lymphocytes profile with low glucose and high protein content can be seen. Cryptococcal meningitis can be recognized early from other meningitis forms with similar lymphocytic CSF profile by simple microscopic examination. A test namely an Indian ink preparation, could be useful. After annexing of a droplet of Indian ink into superset CSF simple and round under light microscope, encapsulated organism appears as bright round bodies among dark background, caused by Indian ink, is the hallmark for definitive diagnosis. It should be notes that *Cryptococcus neoformans* is the most common meningitis in HIV infected patients. Sometimes physicians might diagnosis this condition based on clinical appearance [33].

The recommended treatment for cryptococcal meningitis in HIV infected patients is use of an antifungal drug. The standard therapy of disseminated cryptococcosis--particularly of cerebral manifestation--is still the administration of amphotericin B combined with flucytosine [34 – 39]. Alternative drugs are represented by fluconazole and itraconazole.

However, an azole monotherapy seems to be legitimate only in primary cryptococcosis of the lungs or in early stages of secondary extrapulmonary infection [34 – 39]. Sometimes, chemoprophylaxis for high risk HIV infected cases is used. Out-patient administration of ketoconazole is suggested [40 – 41]. For prevention, it is a rule that an immunocompromised host should not have contact with domestic animals. Control and surveillance of birds as the source of infection is also recommended.

Capillariasis

The nematode (roundworm) *Capillaria philippinensis* is the causative agent of human intestinal capillariasis. It was first discovered in the Philippines in 1963. The life cycle involves freshwater fish as intermediate hosts and fish-eating birds as definitive hosts. Embryonated eggs from feces fed to fish hatch and grow as larvae in the fish intestines. Infective larvae fed to fish-eating birds develop into adults. Larvae become adults in 10 to 11 days, and the first-generation females produce larvae. These larvae develop into males and egg-producing female worms. Eggs pass with the feces, reach water, embryonate, and infect fish. Autoinfection is part of the life cycle and causes hyperinfection. Humans are infected by eating small freshwater fish raw. The parasite multiplies, and symptoms of diarrhea, borborygmus, abdominal pain, and edema develop. Chronic infections lead to malnutrition, malabsorption and hence to protein and electrolyte loss, and death results from irreversible effects of the infection.

In Thailand, the first case report of *Capillaria philippinensis* infection has been published since 1981 by Kunaratanapruk S [42]. Since the first case report, there have been sporadic case reports of the *Capillaria philippinensis* in Thailand. Here, the author performed a literature review on the reports of *Capillaria philippinensis* infections in Thailand in order to summarize the characteristics of this infection among the Thai patients. This study was designed as a descriptive retrospective study. A literature review on the papers concerning *Capillaria philippinensis* infection in Thailand was performed. The author performed the literature review *C. philippinensis* infection reports in Thailand from database of the published works cited in the Index Medicus and Pubmed. The author also reviewed the published works in all 256 local Thai journals, which is not included in the international citation index, for the report of infections in Thailand. The literature review was focused till March 2007. The inclusion criteria consist of the literature as case report of sporadic episode of capillariasis. The exclusion criteria consist of the literature with incomplete data for further analysis. According to the literature review, reports were recruited for further study. The details of clinical presentations of the patients (such as clinical manifestation, diagnosis, treatment and discharge status) in all included reports were studied. The demographic data of all cases including age, sex and address were reviewed as well. Descriptive statistics were used in analyzing the patient characteristics and laboratory parameters for each group. Due to this study, there have been at least 8 reports of *C. philippinensis* infection, of which 1 case was lethal (Table 1). There are at least 12 Thai cases with *C. philippinensis* infections. The age ranges from 13 to 58 years. Of seven well-documented cases, 5 were males and 2 were females. Most (10/12) cases were detected from stool examination: One was detected by

Gastroduodenoscopy: The other case (1/12) was detected after the patient died. Most (11/12) cases had either chronic diarrhea or repeated diarrhea. The antiparasitic drugs were prescribed in most cases Mebendazole in 10 cases and Albendazole in 1 case.

Table 1. Summarization on the cases of patients with capillariasis included in this study

No	Authors	Age (years)	Sex	Address *	diagnosis	Presentation	Treatment	Out come
1	Pathnacharoen et al., 1983[43]	N/A	N/A	NE	Stool examination	Protein – calorie malnutrition	mebendazole 400 mg/day	Cure
2	Pathnacharoen et al., 1983[43]	N/A	N/A	E	Stool examination	Chronic diarrhea with shock	mebendazole 400 mg/day	Cure
3	Pathnacharoen et al., 1983[43]	N/A	N/A	NE	Stool examination	Chronic diarrhea with shock	mebendazole 400 mg/day	Cure
4	Tiensripojamar n et al., 1982[44]	N/A	N/A	C	Stool examination	Chronic diarrhea with malabsorption	mebendazole 400 mg/day	Cure
5	Tiensripojamar n et al., 1982[44]	N/A	N/A	C	Stool examination	Chronic diarrhea with malabsorption	mebendazole 400 mg/day	Cure
6	Tesana et al., 1983[45]	25	Female	NE	Autopsy	Abdominal pain and borborygmi	No	Death
7	Chayakul et al., 1988[46]	58	Male	NE	Stool examination	Chronic diarrhea	mebendazole 400 mg/day	Cure
8	Chayakul et al., 1988[46]	30	Female	NE	Stool examination	Repeated diarrhea and edema	mebendazole 400 mg/day	Cure
9	Chitchang et al., 1979[47]	32	Male	C	Stool examination	Attacks of edema and diarrhea	mebendazole 400 mg/day	Cure
10	Muangmanee et al., 1977[48]	47	Male	NE	Stool examination	6-month history of diarrhea and debility	mebendazole 400 mg/day	Cure
11	Thomnakarn et al., 1998[49]	52	Male	NE	Stool examination	Abdominal pain, chronic diarrhea, malaise	200 mg. of Albendazole	Cure
12	Wongsawasdi et al., 2002[50]	13	Male	C	Gastroduode-noscopy	10-month history of chronic abdominal pain and diarrhea	mebendazole 400 mg/day	Cure

*address is classified according to the Region of Thailand; NE = Northeastern, C = Central

Basically, *Capillaria philippinensis* infection is a nematode infection that occurs most in the Philippines and Thailand. Humans acquire *Capillaria philippinensis* by ingesting of raw or uncooked fish which has infective larvae. The parasite was originally discovered in humans in the Philippines, but since there have also been reports in humans in Thailand C. philippinensis is then considered a zoonotic disease of migratory fish-eating birds. The eggs are disseminated along flyways and infect the fish, and when fish are eaten raw, the disease develops.

Concerning the epidemiology of the patients, the cases can be seen in both sexes and at a wide range of ages. Most reported cases of the infection occurred in the Northeastern region of Thailand. Of interest, Raw food-eating is a deep-rooted eating behavior in Thailand and nearby countries. This traditional eating habit not only brings possible parasitic infection but also allergy [51]. However, it can be seen that there still are documented reported case in the present. This might reflect the unsuccessful attempt in the promotion to not eat uncooked food, in Thailand.

The clinical symptoms and signs found in the patients were similar in all cases. Most patients had diarrhea, abdominal pain, and edema. Few cases had malnutrition, protein–calorie malnutrition. However, there is a fatal case in this series. This case is an infected patient who was pregnant and had a 7-month history of diarrhea after having a 1-month preterm birth the patient had abdominal pain, borborygmi and rapidly lost of weight. The treatment of this case was electrolyte glucose and Sohamin-G replacement. After one day of treatment the patient was dead due to failure of diagnosis. After the autopsy, every stage of *Capillaria philippinensis* was found in the patient's intestine except for its egg. Looking at the 11 cases, who received the antiparasitic treatment, the successful expelling of the parasite could be derived in two ways. First by using mebendazole 400 mg/day, in these cases the period of treatment is about 30 days. Second by using 200 mg. of Albendazole for about 60 days. In conclusion, *Capillaria philippinensis* infection is sporadically reported in Thailand. The diagnosis is usually by stool examination. The survival rate of these infections is high if the diagnosis is correct and is quite low if the diagnosis is too late. The treatment for this infection is an antiparasitic drug such as mebendazole and albendazole [52].

West Nile Encephalitis

West Nile virus infection, a mosquito-borne infection, is a new emerging viral infection. The infection from this virus is caused by a flavivirus transmitted from birds to humans by the bite of culicine mosquitoes [53]. The virus of West Nile was discovered in the blood of a feverish woman of the Western province of Nile in Uganda in 1937 [53]. The West Nile virus can cause the West Nile fever in humans, in a small proportion (around 1 in 150) and the illness can take a severe course associate with symptoms of the central nervous system (encephalitis) and even death, especially in older patients (> 70 years) [53]. While the majority of the humans infected with West Nile virus are asymptomatic, some can develop an influenza-like illness [53]. The caution remains the cornerstone for the recognition and the early control of West Nile virus [53]. The birds serve as the deposit location for the West Nile virus and the virus spreads predominantly by mosquitoes [54]. The mosquitoes of Ornithophilic transmit the virus among bird populations while those species of the mosquito who feed on birds as well as mammals can also transmit the pathogen to humans [54].

Nevertheless, the mammals are considered to be dead ends that do not contribute to the extension of the epidemic of the pathogen [54]. As previously mentioned, the migration of birds has been the important path to diffuse the illnesses of this virus through its history. In the Western hemisphere, the infection of this virus has been diagnosed and has been mentioned for its relation to the migration of infected birds from endemic areas in recent years. Humans, horses, birds, and vector mosquito are the important components of the infection. The West Nile virus is an important arthropod –borne flavivirus; it generally causes a temperate infection called the West Nile fever in the humans and horses. The mosquitoes are the main vectors of West Nile virus [55]. Several species of Culex is found to act as vectors in different geographical regions [55]. The experimental studies had shown that *Culex triataeniorhynchus*, *Culex vishnui*, *Culex bitaeniorhynchus* and *Culex univittatus*, *Culex pipiens fatigans* and *Aedes albopictus* would be able to act as potential vectors of West Nile virus [55].

There are some recent interesting reports in the epidemiology of the West Nile virus infection. Recently, Peterson et al. utilized a shaping study to investigate the spreading of the infection of this virus in the US [56]. They found that the situation with mosquitoes did not coincide with guidelines observed of the extension, while the other with mosquitoes and migratory birds coincided suggesting that the guidelines observed for the extension were explained better with migratory birds, agents of long distance, as the critics of transportation; the virus, in regions to which it had been transported by migratory birds, then was transmitted enzootically to mosquitoes [56]. Brownstein et al. carried out another spatial analysis of West Nile virus for the evaluation of the risk of a vector-borne introduced zoonosis [57]. They found that that logistic regression analysis revealed satellite-derived vegetation to be significantly and positively strong association with the presence of human cases [57]. Besides the broadcast owing to thevector, other ways the West Nile virus spread are also mentioned. In animals, Banet-Noach et al. totally suggested that horizontal broadcast of West Nile virus would be able to occur in commercial multitudes and might be aggravated if the cannibalism and feather-choosing of sick geese occurred [58]. The new ways of the broadcast by contributions of blood, by transplants of organ, and by the intrauterine routes have also been reported. The possible broadcast of the mother to infant through breast milk is also mentioned [59]. Some pregnant women can also be susceptible to the virus and if they experience the infection, the vertical broadcast of West Nile virus infection to their infants can be expected. The intrapartum infection of West Nile virus is interesting in obstetrics. A report that describes a case of transplacental West Nile transmission was noted in 2002 [59]. It is noted that pregnant women should take the precautions to reduce its risk for the West Nile virus or another infection of arboviral group and should experience to test when clinically appropriates [59]. In 2003, Alpert et al. said that intrauterine broadcast of West Nile virus might have as a result the significant morbidity of ocular and neurological systems [60]. They noted that the titers for this important pathogen should be obtained when standard serology was refused in a boy with congenital markings of chorioretinal organ [60]. In 2004, Central for Illnesses Controls and Prevention (CDC) proposed provisional guidelines for the evaluation of children born to mothers infected with West Nile virus [61]. During 2002, CDC investigated 3 cases of the maternal West Nile virus infection and found that the children were born full term with normal appearance and negative laboratory tests of for the virus infection [61]. In 2002, CDC also proposed for a case of possible spreading of the virus to a boy by breast-feeding [62]. In this case, the boy was exposed to the mother's milk and found to have West Nile virus by TaqMan molecular test [63].

The infections in humans are generally asymptomatic. The most serious demonstration of the infection is encephalitis in humans and horses, as well as mortality in birds. Recently, nevertheless, a growing number of cases that imply the demonstrations of central nervous system and death have been reported in people of advanced age. The fever, pains of general parts of the body, headache, nausea and vomiting were the main clinical characteristics in 90% of the hospitalized cases [64]. The treatment process for the West Nile virus infection should be based on the severity of the infection. Similar to the general viral infection, the specific methods are not available for the processing of the West Nile virus infection. Since most cases with West Nile virus infections are temperate, no intensive treatment is needed in those non - severe cases. Nevertheless, supporting therapy is recommended for the patients with encephalitis. There are some recent reports on the possible antiviral drugs for the infection. Morrey et al. recently carried out a study in the culture of the cell and in the rodent the animal models to determine the efficacy of interferon-alpha (IFN-alpha), the interferon (IFN) inducers and ribavirin, alone or in the combination with IFN, to treat West Nile virus [64].

Psittacosis

Psittacosis is an important chlmmydial infection. *Chlamydia psittaci* is the etiological agent. Eidson said that decreasing imports of birds and increasing education might contribute to a reduction in human risk from avian infections [65]. Eidson also noted that keeping new birds separate from old birds in aviaries and poultry production facilities might reduce the incidence of avian chlamydiosis [65]. Psittacosis is a relatively common cause of community acquired pneumonia in adults [66]. Although the illness is usually mild to moderate in severity, it can be life threatening. It should be considered as a possible cause of any flu-like illness [67]. Parrots and other psittacine birds still are regarded as the major reservoir of the infectious agent, and most recognized cases are associated with owning pet birds or working in a pet store [68 - 69]. The diagnosis frequently is first considered in evaluating a patient whose pneumonia has not responded to therapy with a beta-lactam antibiotic [69 – 69]. It is concluded that the diagnosis of avian chlamydiosis is laborious and that there is still a need for more accurate, simple and rapid diagnostic tools, both for antigen and antibody detection in various species of birds [70]. A targeted therapy for diseases in humans and birds is successfully possible with chlortetracycline, doxycycline or fluoroquinolone-containing drugs. The diagnosis usually is established serologically [68]. The clinical diagnosis of psittacosis can be made early usually, particularly in the presence of pneumonitis on a chest x-ray film and a positive history of bird contact [71]. Tetracycline or doxycycline is the preferred therapy and is administered for three weeks to prevent relapses [68]. Treatment with doxycycline (100 mg twice a day for 14 days) is recommended [72 – 74]. Similar to other bird - borne diseases, avoidance of bird contact is a good basic preventive method for psittacosis [72 - 74]. Kaleta et al. suggested that government-imposed control measures focusing entirely on imported psittacines such as quarantine, long-term medication and possibly eradication of Chlamydia psittaci-positive psittacine birds were not essential any more [75].

References

[1]   Steele JH. Occupational health in agriculture. Animal-borne diseases. *Arch. Environ. Health.* 1968 Aug;17(2):267-85.

[2]   Grimes JE. Zoonoses acquired from pet birds. *Vet Clin North Am Small Anim Pract.* 1987 Jan;17(1):209-18.

[3]   Warnock DW. Fungal diseases: an evolving public health challenge. *Ed. Mycol.* 2006 Dec;44(8):697-705.

[4]   Zhou Q, Murphy WJ. Immune response and immunotherapy to Cryptococcus infections. *Immunol. Res.* 2006;35(3):191-208.

[5]   Okabayashi K, Hasegawa A, Watanabe T. Microreview: capsule-associated genes of Cryptococcus neoformans. *Mycopathologia.* 2007 Jan;163(1):1-8.

[6]   Chayakulkeeree M, Perfect JR. Cryptococcosis. *Infect. Dis. Clin. North Am.* 2006 Sep;20(3):507-44, v-vi.

[7]   Hoang LM, Maguire JA, Doyle P, Fyfe M, Roscoe DL. Cryptococcus neoformans infections at Vancouver Hospital and Health Sciences Centre (1997-2002): epidemiology, microbiology and histopathology. *J. Med. Microbiol.* 2004 Sep;53(Pt 9):935-40.

[8]   Banerjee U, Datta K, Majumdar T, Gupta K. Cryptococcosis in India: the awakening of a giant? *Med. Mycol.* 2001 Feb;39(1):51-67.

[9]   de Melo NT, Lacaz Cda S, Charbel CE, Pereira AD, Heins-Vaccari EM, Franca-Netto AS, Machado Ldos R, Livramento JA. Cryptococcus neoformans chemotyping. Review of the literature. New epidemiologic data on cryptococcosis. Our experience with the use of C.G.B. media in the study of this yeast. *Rev. Inst. Med. Trop. Sao Paulo.* 1993 Sep-Oct;35(5):469-78.

[10]   Malik R, Krockenberger MB, Cross G, Doneley R, Madill DN, Black D, McWhirter P, Rozenwax A, Rose K, Alley M, Forshaw D, Russell-Brown I, Johnstone AC, Martin P, O'Brien CR, Love DN. Avian cryptococcosis. *Med. Mycol.* 2003 Apr;41(2):115-24.

[11]   Blaschke-Hellmessen R. Cryptococcus species--etiological agents of zoonoses or sapronosis? *Mycoses.* 2000;43 Suppl 1:48-60.

[12]   Perfect JR. Cryptococcus neoformans: the yeast that likes it hot. *FEMS Yeast Res.* 2006 Jun;6(4):463-8.

[13]   Lin X, Heitman J. The biology of the Cryptococcus neoformans species complex. *Annu. Rev. Microbiol.* 2006;60:69-105.

[14]   Hull CM, Heitman J. Genetics of Cryptococcus neoformans. *Annu. Rev. Genet.* 2002;36:557-615.

[15]   Ellis D, Pfeiffer T. The ecology of Cryptococcus neoformans. *Eur. J. Epidemiol.* 1992 May;8(3):321-5.

[16] Ellis DH, Pfeiffer TJ. Ecology, life cycle, and infectious propagule of Cryptococcus neoformans. *Lancet.* 1990 Oct 13;336(8720):923-5.

[17] Soogarun S, Wiwanitkit V, Palasuwan A, Pradniwat P, Suwansaksri J, Lertlum T, Maungkote T. Detection of Cryptococcus neoformans in bird excreta. *Southeast Asian J. Trop. Med. Public Health.* 2006 Jul;37(4):768-70.

[18] Kielstein P, Hotzel H, Schmalreck A, Khaschabi D, Glawischnig W. Occurrence of Cryptococcus spp. in excreta of pigeons and pet birds. *Mycoses.* 2000;43(1-2):7-15.

[19] Kohno S. Clinical and mycological features of cryptococcosis. *Nippon Ishinkin Gakkai Zasshi.* 2003;44(3):159-62.

[20] Machnicka-Rowinska B. Parasitoses in immune deficiencies. *Wiad Parazytol.* 2000;46(3):335-44.

[21] Chakrabarti A. Microbiology of systemic fungal infections. *J. Postgrad Med.* 2005;51 Suppl. 1:S16-20.

[22] Mitchell TG, Perfect JR. Cryptococcosis in the era of AIDS--100 years after the discovery of Cryptococcus neoformans. *Clin. Microbiol. Rev.* 1995 Oct;8(4):515-48.

[23] Waters L, Nelson M. Cryptococcal disease and HIV infection. *Expert Opin. Pharmacother.* 2005 Dec;6(15):2633-44.

[24] Haddad NE, Powderly WG. The changing face of mycoses in patients with HIV/AIDS. *AIDS Read.* 2001 Jul;11(7):365-8, 375-8

[25] Manfredi R, Pieri F, Pileri SA, Chiodo F. The changing face of AIDS-related opportunism: cryptococcosis in the highly active antiretroviral therapy (HAART) era. Case reports and literature review. *Mycopathologia.* 1999 Nov;148(2):73-8.

[26] Mitchell TG, Perfect JR. Cryptococcosis in the era of AIDS--100 years after the discovery of Cryptococcus neoformans. *Clin. Microbiol. Rev.* 1995 Oct;8(4):515-48.

[27] Corr P. Imaging of neuro-AIDS. *J. Psychosom. Res.* 2006 Sep;61(3):295-9.

[28] Trujillo JR, Jaramillo Rangel G, Ortega-Martinez M, Penalva de Oliveira AC, Vidal JE, Bryant J, Gallo RC. International NeuroAIDS: prospects of HIV-1 associated neurological complications. *Cell Res.* 2005 Nov-Dec;15(11-12):962-9. Review

[29] Malinverni R, Furrer H. CNS-infections in HIV patients. *Ther Umsch.* 1999 Nov;56(11):670-4.

[30] Kishida S. Neurological manifestations associated with HIV-1 infection] *No To Shinkei.* 1997 Jan;49(1):25-37.

[31] Bicanic T, Harrison TS. Cryptococcal meningitis. *Br Med Bull.* 2005 Apr 18;72:99-118.

[32] del Brutto OH. Central nervous system mycotic infections. *Rev. Neurol.* 2000 Mar 1-15;30(5):447-59.

[33] Subramanian S, Mathai D. Clinical manifestations and management of cryptococcal infection. *J. Postgrad. Med.* 2005;51 Suppl 1:S21-6.

[34] Berenguer Berenguer J. Commonly used antifungal agents in the treatment of systemic mycoses. *Rev. Clin. Esp.* 1995 Oct;195 Suppl 3:58-65

[35] Graybill JR. The future of antifungal therapy. *Clin. Infect. Dis.* 1996 May;22 Suppl 2:S166-78

[36] Sarosi GA, Davies SF. Therapy for fungal infections. *Mayo Clin. Proc.* 1994 Nov;69(11):1111-7.

[37] Stevens DA. Therapy for opportunistic fungal infections: past, present and future. *Indian J. Cancer.* 1995 Mar;32(1):1-9.

[38] Yonga G. Current drug therapy of systemic mycoses: a review. *East Afr. Med. J.* 1995 Jun;72(6):394-8.

[39] Just-Nubling G. Therapy of candidiasis and cryptococcosis in AIDS. *Mycoses.* 1994;37 Suppl. 2:56-63.

[40] Terrell CL. Antifungal agents. Part II. The azoles. *Mayo Clin. Proc.* 1999 Jan;74(1):78-100.

[41] Como JA, Dismukes WE. Oral azole drugs as systemic antifungal therapy. *N. Engl. J. Med.* 1994 Jan 27;330(4):263-72.

[42] Kunaratanapruk S, Iam-Ong S, Chatsirimongkol C. Intestinal capillariasis. *Ramathibodi Med. J.* 1981; 4 : 206 – 13.

[43] Pathnacharoen S, Tansuphaswadikul S, Manutstitt S, Thanangkul B. *Intestinal capillariasis Ramathibodi. Med. J.* 1983; 6: 277 – 83

[44] Tiensripojamarn A, Jarajinda S, Veerakula K, Rutapichairuxa N. *R. Thai Air Force Med. Gaz.*1982; 28: 193 – 7

[45] Tesana S, Bhuripanyo K, Sanpitak P, Sithithaworn P. Intestinal capillariasis from Udon Thani Province, Northeastern part of Thailand. *J. Med. Assoc. Thai* 1983; 66: 128 – 31

[46] Chayakul P, Ovartlarnporn B, Kulwichit P, Piratvisut T, Kunasakdakun A. Intestinal capillariasis. *J. Infect. Dis. Antimicrob. Agents* 1988; 5: 187 – 90

[47] Chitchang S, Chitprasong T, JanTong T, Suksala N. Intestinal capillariasis from Lopburi Province. *R. Thai Army Med. J.* 1979; 32: 163 – 5

[48] Muangmanee L, Aswapokee N, Vanasin B. Intestinal capillariasis. *Siriraj Hosp Gaz* 1977; 29: 439 – 45

[49] Thomnakarn K, Penpinich C, Saietang S. Intestinal capillariasis at Khon Kaen Regional Hospital. *Khon Kaen Hosp Med J* 1998; 22: 65 – 7

[50] Wongsawasdi L, Ukarapol N, Lertprasertsuk N. The endoscopic diagnosis of intestinal capillariasis in a child. *Southeast Asian J. Trop. Med. Public Health.* 2002 Dec;33(4):730 – 2

[51] Pitetti RD, Kuspis D, Krenzelok EP. Caterpillars: an unusual source of ingestion. *Pediatr Emerg Care* 1999;15:33-6.

[52] Cross JH, Basaca-Sevilla V. Intestinal capillariasis. *Prog Clin Parasitol.* 1989;1:105-19.

[53] Guharoy R, Gilroy SA, Noviasky JA, Ference J. West Nile virus infection. *Am. J. Health Syst. Pharm.* 2004; 61: 1235-41.

[54] Pauli G. West Nile virus. Prevalence and significance as a zoonotic pathogen. *Bundesgesundheitsblatt. Gesundheitsforschung. Gesundheitsschutz.* 2004; 47: 653-60.

[55] Paramasivan R, Mishra AC, Mourya DT. West Nile virus: the Indian scenario. *Indian J. Med. Res.* 2003; 118:101-8.

[56] Peterson AT, Vieglais DA, Andreasen JK. Migratory birds modeled as critical transport agents for West Nile Virus in North America. *Vector Borne Zoonotic Dis.* 2003; 3: 27-37.

[57] Banet-Noach C, Simanov L, Malkinson M. Direct (non-vector) transmission of West Nile virus in geese. *Avian Pathol.* 2003; 32: 489-94.

[58] Intrauterine West Nile virus infection--New York, 2002. MMWR. Morb. *Mortal Wkly Rep.* 2002; 51: 1135-6.

[59] Alpert SG, Fergerson J, Noel LP. Intrauterine West Nile virus: ocular and systemic findings. *Am. J. Ophthalmol.* 2003; 136: 733-5.

[60] Center for Diseases Control and Prevention (CDC). Interim guidelines for the evaluation of infants born to mothers infected with West Nile virus during pregnancy. *MMWR Morb. Mortal Wkly Rep.* 2004; 53: 154-7.

[61] From the Centers for Disease Control and Prevention. Possible West Nile virus transmission to an infant through breast-feeding--Michigan, 2002. *JAMA.* 2002; 288: 1976-7.

[62] Possible West Nile virus transmission to an infant through breast-feeding--Michigan, 2002. *MMWR Morb Mortal Wkly Rep.* 2002; 51: 877-8

[63] Center for Diseases Control and Prevention (CDC). Transfusion-associated transmission of West Nile virus--Arizona, 2004. *MMWR Morb. Mortal Wkly Rep.* 2004; 53: 842-4.

[64] Thakare JP, Rao TL, Padbidri VS. Prevalence of West Nile virus infection in India. *Southeast Asian J. Trop. Med. Public Health.* 2002; 33: 801-5

[65] Morrey JD, Day CW, Julander JG, Blatt LM, Smee DF, Sidwell RW. Effect of interferon-alpha and interferon-inducers on West Nile virus in mouse and hamster animal models. *Antivir Chem Chemother.* 2004; 15: 101-9.

[66] Eidson M. Psittacosis/avian chlamydiosis. *J. Am. Vet. Med. Assoc.* 2002 Dec 15;221(12):1710-2.

[67] Elliott JH. Psittacosis. A flu like syndrome. *Aust Fam Physician.* 2001 Aug;30(8):739-41

[68] Gregory DW, Schaffner W. Psittacosis. *Semin. Respir. Infect.* 1997 Mar;12(1):7-11.

[69] Kirchner JT. Psittacosis. Is contact with birds causing your patient's pneumonia? *Postgrad. Med.* 1997 Aug;102(2):181-2, 187-8, 193-4.

[70] Vanrompay D, Ducatelle R, Haesebrouck F. Chlamydia psittaci infections: a review with emphasis on avian chlamydiosis. *Vet. Microbiol.* 1995 Jul;45(2-3):93-119.

[71] Yung AP, Grayson ML. Psittacosis--a review of 135 cases. *Med. J. Aust.* 1988 Mar 7;148(5):228-33.

[72] Johnston WB, Eidson M, Smith KA, Stobierski MG. Compendium of chlamydiosis (psittacosis) control, 1999. Psittacosis Compendium Committee, National Association of State Public Health Veterinarians. *J.Am .Vet. Med. Assoc.* 1999 Mar 1;214(5):640-6.

[73] Sachse K, Grossmann E. Chlamydial diseases of domestic animals--zoonotic potential of the agents and diagnostic issues. *Dtsch Tierarztl Wochenschr.* 2002 Apr;109(4):142-8.

[74] Macfarlane JT, Macrae AD. Psittacosis. *Br.Med.Bull.* 1983 Apr;39(2):163-7.

[75] Kaleta EF, Krautwald-Junghanns ME, Redmann T. Psittacosis (chlamydiosis) of birds and the necessity of government disease control. *Tierarztl Prax Ausg K Klientiere Heimtiere.* 1998 Jul;26(4):295-301.

Index

B

G

H

I

T

U

V

virology, xv, 79, 100, 134

virus infection, xiii, xviii, 6, 23, 31, 32, 36, 37, 39, 40, 43, 51, 53, 59, 60, 61, 63, 72, 74, 80, 85, 87, 88, 98, 103, 108, 109, 110, 113, 117, 145, 146, 147, 150, 151

virus replication, 53, 57

vomiting, 52, 55, 106, 147

vRNA, vii

vulnerability, 135, 142

W

Wales, xiv, 137

war, 35, 50, 123

Washington, x, 35, 135

waste disposal, 100

water vapor, 123

waterfowl, x, xii, 16, 20, 22, 24, 36, 47, 102, 122

weak interaction, 68

weakness, 52

wear, 92, 96

web, 65

web service, 65

weight loss, 52

welfare, 117, 136

West Nile fever, 145

West Nile virus, 146, 147, 150, 151

Western countries, 31

Western Hemisphere, xvi

Western Siberia, 43, 48

wheezing, 108

wholesale, 16

wild type, 107

wildlife, xi

wind, 93

winter, 10, 22, 73

Wisconsin, 118

women, 116, 123, 146

work absenteeism, 138

workers, 28, 34, 96, 115, 116, 121, 123, 124, 130, 132

World Health Organization (WHO), viii, 4, 10, 11, 22, 30, 35, 37, 58, 73, 99, 111, 117, 121, 126, 133

worms, 143

X

X-ray, 10, 27, 107, 147

Y

yawning, xiv

yeast, 142, 148

yolk, xi, 94

Z

zinc, 92

zoonosis, 12, 71, 146

zoonotic, 21, 72, 139, 145, 150, 151